SEXPLORATION

Jane Bogart is a nationally known "sexpert." She has appeared on MTV's *First National Sex Quiz* and *True Life: I Need a Sex Rx*. Currently, she is the Coordinator of Student Health Outreach and Promotion (SHOP) at the University of California Santa Cruz (UCSC). For the previous ten years, she was Director of Health Promotion at New York University, where students nicknamed her "Sex Jane." At UCSC, she is responsible for outreach, education, and prevention around issues related to sexuality and sexual health, alcohol and other drugs, eating, stress and smoking, and holistic health concerns. She was the recipient of NYU's Outstanding Faculty/Staff Service to the Lesbian, Gay, Bisexual and Transgender Community Award.

Bogart teaches Human Sexuality Education and Social Marketing at Columbia University, is chair-elect for the Health Promotion Section of the American College Health Association, serves as a consultant for the Kaiser Family Foundation, and has been a trainer with the United Nations Population Fund in Eastern Europe. She has a master's degree in health education from Teachers College, Columbia University, and is a Certified Health Education Specialist, a rape crisis counselor, and an HIV pre- and post-test counselor. She lives in Santa Cruz, California, with her twenty-eight-pound cat, Pooh.

SEXPLORATION

* * *

SEXPLORATION

***

The Ultimate Guide to Feeling Truly Great in Bed

***

Written and Illustrated by

JANE BOGART, MA, CHES

Additional writing and research by Ellen Friedrichs, MA

PENGUIN BOOKS

PENGUIN BOOKS

Published by the Penguin Group

Penguin Group (USA) Inc., 375 Hudson Street, New York, New York 10014, U.S.A.
Penguin Group (Canada), 90 Eglinton Avenue East, Suite 700, Toronto, Ontario,
Canada M4P 2Y3 (a division of Pearson Penguin Canada Inc.)
Penguin Books Ltd, 80 Strand, London WC2R 0RL, England
Penguin Ireland, 25 St Stephen's Green, Dublin 2, Ireland
(a division of Penguin Books Ltd)
Penguin Group (Australia), 250 Camberwell Road, Camberwell, Victoria 3124, Australia
(a division of Pearson Australia Group Pty Ltd)
Penguin Books India Pvt Ltd, 11 Community Centre, Panchsheel Park,
New Delhi – 110 017, India
Penguin Group (NZ), cnr Airborne and Rosedale Roads, Albany, Auckland 1310,
New Zealand (a division of Pearson New Zealand Ltd)
Penguin Books (South Africa) (Pty) Ltd, 24 Sturdee Avenue, Rosebank,
Johannesburg 2196, South Africa

Penguin Books Ltd, Registered Offices:
80 Strand, London WC2R 0RL, England

First published in Penguin Books 2006

1   3   5   7   9   10   8   6   4   2

Copyright © Jane Bogart, 2006
All rights reserved

LIBRARY OF CONGRESS CATALOGING IN PUBLICATION DATA
Bogart, Jane, date.
Sexploration : the ultimate guide to feeling truly great in bed / Jane Bogart.
p.   cm.
ISBN 0-14-303685-8
1. Sex instruction.   2. Sex.   3. Sex (Psychology)   I. Title.
HQ31.B5934   2006
613.9'6—dc22   2005052781

Printed in the United States of America
Set in Bembo
Designed by Mia Risberg

For Dinah Bogart

Contents

✳ Contents ✳

✳ *Acknowledgments* ✳

Whenever I get a new book, I turn first to the acknowledgments page because it gives me some sense of who the author is as a person and what is important to her or him. I have always fantasized about being able to write acknowledgments in my own book, and now that I have that opportunity, I find myself a bit stymied by the task. As I look back over my turbulent, quixotic, and unfinished life, I find that an overwhelming number of people have supported and guided me in my journey. Following are just some of those to whom I owe gratitude.

First and foremost, I thank the three wise women who are my constant support system: Johanna Soet, my chosen soul sister and fellow feisty girl—I can't imagine my life without you; Glori Bine, cherished friend, who is my rock and voice of reason and who lives her life so admirably; and Jane Bowman (the other Jane) without whom I just wouldn't have survived the ups and downs of the past eleven years.

My colleagues at NYU for allowing me to bloom, take chances, and make mistakes and for providing a compassionate ear, particularly Todd Smith, Bob Butler, Stephen Polniaszek, David Vogelsang, Yolanda Cacciolo, Marianna Zane, Susan Schlesiona, Susan Orand, Phyllis LaMonaca, Alfred Giosa, Don Kreuz, Carlo Ciotoli (miss me yet?), Jennie Tichenor, Nancy Young, Patty Delorenzo, Fred Cohen, and the members of the AMC.

My new colleagues at UCSC—Sherri Sobin, Tammy Wood,

Diane Lamotte, Les Elkind, Gerry Gerringer, Robert Antonino, Eleanor Gillis, and Paul Willis, who have welcomed me with enthusiastic open arms. To Meg Kobe and Michael Dorenzo for being incredibly talented and collaborative.

All of the phenomenal students at NYU and UCSC who continue to inspire me in unimaginable ways. Special thanks to Keeley, Chelsea, Ian, Miriam and Kendra, Claudia, Ken, Phillip, Guido, Becky, and Patty.

My fellow health promotion professionals and friends—it is an honor to work with and learn from you—Bob Ward, Jane Emmeree, Cathy Kodama, Michelle Johnston, Jenny Haubenreiser, Sarah Mart, Jordan Friedman, Carole Pertofsky, Paula Swinford, Pam Viele, Sabina White, Billie Lindsey, and Pat Fabiano.

Toni Mufson and Steve Goldstein for their unerring wisdom and guidance through the murky depths of life and relationships.

Judith Steinhart for being an inspiring sexuality educator, mentor, and friend; Francesca Maresca (and Deb) for teaching me so much about education and social justice and friendship; Kurt Zischke, my first husband, lifelong friend, and truly enlightened man (and his wife, Tori), for unwavering support and belief in me.

I am also grateful to the following people: Martin Fetner for the years of friendship, Michael Owens for believing in and encouraging my dancing, Norma Smith and Sally Broido for generously sharing their lives with me, Rachel Wineberg for hanging in there all of these years, Joey Blumenthal for being there, Ken Resnicow for helping when I needed him, Noah and Gabriel Resnicow for lighting up my life, Mike, Michael, Amanda, and Gabriella Callagy, Debra Linden for remaining a bastion of sanity and getting me David Cassidy's autograph, Maddie Holzer for living a life to which I can aspire, Catherine Charlton for giving me the opportunity to begin a new career, Mike Livanos for propelling me into the healing place I needed to be, Annette Huelett for new skills and insight, Howell Wechsler for so much, Felicia Brabec for reading and editing and encouraging, Donald Sheehan, Robert Zenie, Brian Paquette, Bill Coury, Geralyn Coopersmith, Lori Ende, Jose Nanin, Nancy Goldberg, and my cousins Jane and Pete Doft and Ellen and Jerome Stern.

Jen Barefoot for recommending me to the Kaiser Family Foundation, which began this fantastic exploration; Julia Davis and Tina Hoff at Kaiser Family Foundation for believing in my capabilities; the folks at MTV who took a chance on me; Jane Dystel and Miriam Goderich, my wonderful agents and cheerleaders, and Brett Kelly, my fantastic editor at Penguin Books.

Ellen Friedrichs, sexuality educator and writer par excellence, without whom this book would not have been completed. Her research, writing, and intelligent insights helped drive *Sexploration*.

Finally, I am grateful to the members of my family: my father for his kindness, humor, and love; my wonderful stepmother, Dorothy, for her unwavering support, empathetic ear, and confidence in my ability; my brother, Gary, for being my biggest fan, strongest defender, and companion in life's adventures; and my stepsiblings, Jodi and Wayne Ballard and Paul and Nicole Ginsberg, and my nieces and nephews for the best kinship genetics can't buy.

What Is Sexploration?

*That the ability to copulate is not clinically a meaningful
indicator of much of anything has not shaken people's belief that
if they can fuck they are fine: they are judged healthy, with all
that implies about the fulfillment of life.*
—Stuart Schneiderman, *Jaques Lacan*

I'm not going to make any assumptions about you and sex.
Maybe you've never had sex with another person or
you've had a lot of sex with many different people. Maybe you
love sex, or you hate sex, or you're pretty neutral about it.
Maybe you know a lot about sex, or maybe you're still trying to
figure out where the heck the clitoris is. Maybe you've had
wonderful, passionate encounters, or maybe you've had traumatic, confusing, or dissatisfying experiences fraught with fum-
bling and missteps. Hey, maybe you're having sex right now.

I'm here to tell you that there is no perfect sex life. Human
behavior around sex is unpredictable because your body and
your mind are both fallible. People are not machines. Normal
human sexuality encompasses a wide range of activities, feelings,
and experiences. To make it more complicated, sexuality is dynamic, not static, which means that who you are as a sexual human being will change over the course of your life. How your

body responds sexually, your sexual likes and dislikes, your feelings about sexuality, and your interest level in sexual activity can change from day to day.

The other catch is that sex often involves other people, so it's not just your sexual stuff that you have to contend with; it's their stuff, too. One person's turn-on can be another's turn-off. It's rare to find two people who are magically sexually compatible, and even when you do, it's not uncommon for one of you to be in the mood while the other wants nothing more than to go to sleep. That's life. That's sex.

And that's where *Sexploration* comes in. *Sexploration* is a practical, human, and humorous sexuality guide that will supply you with accurate, compelling information, interactive, thoughtful exercises and activities, and shared anecdotes to help you figure out for yourself where you've been, where you are, and where you'd like to go on your sexual journey through life. You can be comfortable with your body, be at home with your desires, communicate with your partner(s), and really, truly enjoy yourself in bed—or *out of bed,* whatever the case may be.

By examining your sexual attitudes, values, and beliefs and knowing, exploring, and challenging your own limits and boundaries, you will come closer to the sex life that's best for you. You will learn how to adapt to the twists, turns, bumps, and other unexpected changes that are inevitable in your sexual journey.

My own sexual journey has been peppered with both foibles and fantastic adventures. It's what makes me human. In my work as a sexuality educator, I've found that sharing experiences, stories, and information is one of the most enlightening ways to learn. This doesn't often happen with sexuality. But throughout this book you'll find stories from others, both similar and dissimilar to your experiences, that can help you expand your concept of sexuality and direct your sexual journeys.

Each one of us is different, and I won't make generalizations or tell you what I think you should do. I am not you; I do not live your life, and I certainly don't know what's best for you. There are no rules; it is most important to do what makes sense for you. Read and use the parts of this book that you are comfortable using, and try to push yourself a bit out of your comfort zone so that you can grow. If certain activities or suggestions make you anxious, skip them or go back to them when you feel ready.

Embarking on a sexploration isn't necessarily simple. It involves challenging yourself to grow, to try different ways of interacting and talking about sex. It involves asking yourself—and perhaps learning how to ask others—questions that may not be readily answered, questions with and without right and wrong answers, and perhaps even questions to which you thought you knew the answers. It involves confronting your judgments and

A NOTE FOR SURVIVORS OF SEXUAL VIOLENCE

This book is for anyone who is interested in exploring his or her sexuality regardless of age, sex, gender identity, sexual orientation, or survivor status; however, it is not intended as a guide for coming to terms with the effects of past sexual violence (such as childhood sexual abuse, sexual assault, or rape). If you are a survivor of sexual violence who is just embarking on your healing journey, I encourage you to seek additional resources and assistance in coming to understand and heal from the effects your past experience may have had on your current sexual self. There are several books on this topic listed in the resources section. Professional help in the form of a trained therapist who specializes in sexual violence is also an invaluable resource for anyone who is struggling with these issues.

assumptions and working through your anxieties. And it involves practice!

Here are five guiding principles I think are most important to keep in mind:*

- Sexuality is a positive, life-affirming force. The ultimate goal is for you to have fun and feel good!
- Sex is more than sexual intercourse and should be more than orgasm goal oriented. Sexuality involves taste and smell and touch and sound. There are many, *many* ways to be sexual without penetration. By broadening your definition of sex, you can alleviate many of your sexual problems and concerns, expand your sexual repertoire, and improve your loving.
- People vary in their comfort level with sexual language, sexual behavior, and sexual risk taking. Language, especially language around sexuality, has meaning, and those meanings differ from person to person—my curse word may be your word of endearment; one woman's "vagina" may be another's "down there," and one man's "penis" may be another man's "shlong."
- Learning about sexuality is a lifelong adventure. Sexuality begins at birth and ends with death.
- Normal sexuality encompasses a wide range of expression, including sexual orientation, gender identity, sexual experience, ethnic identity, and sexual practice.

---

* Some of these guidelines are adapted from Peggy Brick and Jan Lunquist, *New Expectations: Sexuality Education for Mid and Later Life* (New York: SIECUS, 2003).

It is not the ultimate goal of this book to make you into some physically programmed sex god/goddess/robot. This book is not about mastering specific techniques. This book is not about achieving "the ultimate orgasm" or the art of maintaining a five-hour erection. This book is about you. It's about helping you understand your sexual journey up to this point in time and to help you map out a course for the future so that you feel happy and healthy and comfortable enough to have the ultimate orgasm or understand why you may or may not be interested in maintaining a five-hour erection. It's about uncovering your sexual longings, talking about them with your partner, and learning how to give and receive pleasure in a way that makes you feel fantastic. Because after all, that is what it means to be truly "great in bed."

SEXPLORATION

* * *

Chapter 1

THE JOURNEY BEGINS

Starting Your Sexploration

* * *

> *For there are three elements that contribute to sexual functioning—knowledge, comfort and choice . . . and they are interlocking, mutually reinforcing elements. To know is one thing; to be comfortable with what one knows is another; to choose what is right for oneself is still another.*
> —Masters and Johnson

*W*ander into your neighborhood bookstore and peruse the travel section. No matter where you choose to go, you'll find many books to guide you in your travels. Why? Because it makes sense to know where you're going before you get there. At minimum, you want to have some idea of the culture, the climate, the currency used, and the basics on how to get around so you can be comfortable. Otherwise you may end up in a place like Reykjavík, Iceland, in the middle of winter, wearing shorts, a T-shirt, and flip-flops, squinting through your Ray-Bans, a wallet full of shekels, looking for the subway. (If you've never been to Iceland, I assure you that Reykjavík, although beautiful, is cold and very, very dark in the winter, you can't buy anything with shekels, and there is definitely no subway system.)

You may at times be traveling solo, but you will most likely have a traveling companion, or two, or three. If you've ever traveled with someone else, you know that his or her quirks can make or break your trip. There's nothing more disconcerting than finding out that you're with a "plan every second of the day, get up early, visit every museum, stick to the itinerary" person when you are a "spontaneous, fly by the seat of your pants, let's see where this road takes us" voyager. Bottom line—you want to be prepared for your journey. Or, as my mother used to say, "You want to make sure you have clean underwear!"

It's the same with sexuality. You may be primed to jump right in ("Get out the handcuffs and slather me with lubricant—yahoo!"), or you may want to take a more tentative approach ("Don't expect me to stray too far from that old faithful missionary position"). Trying new things and new ways of doing old things can evoke both excitement and apprehension. In *Sexploration,* there are opportunities for both ends of the adventure spectrum and the entire range in between.

That's necessary because, much like the weather, our bodies and our sexual desires and needs are constantly evolving and changing, ebbing and flowing and responding. Any change in your life—ending or starting a relationship, an illness or disability (whether temporary or chronic), stress (and who doesn't have this in his or her life), gaining or losing weight, having children, even having a bad day—affects our sexual needs and desires.

If you have a longtime companion or spouse, it is likely that he or she will also go through changes over the course of your time together. If you start a new relationship, you will have to adjust and adapt to another person's needs and wants, which are most likely to be different from your previous partner's needs and wants, not to mention your own.

Like any other excursion, a sexploration requires predeparture planning. You need to figure out the "lay of the land" (so to speak) to guarantee that your sexual journey with yourself and your partners is safe and exciting. But the truth is that we seldom prepare sufficiently for our sexual journeys, and then we wonder how the heck we are so unequipped for the place and person (or persons) with whom we have ended up.

This book is not going to help you achieve the perfect sex life, because (let's be serious) nobody has the perfect anything. But it will help you challenge yourself within your own limitations, give you tools to address particular situations, communicate your needs, negotiate with partners who have different turn-ons from your own, confront your personal inhibitions, expand your definition of sex, and teach you new ways of sexual pleasuring. It can help you identify which of your sexual behaviors are healthy and which are sexually hindering—so that you can be truly great in bed, whatever that entails or means to you.

If you've had negative or disappointing experiences around sex, you might feel you need to do some type of work on that. If you are ashamed of or not comfortable with your body, you may want to work on improving your body image as your goal. Part of a sexploration is setting the parameters within which you can safely explore. Following are some of the guidelines I have found to be helpful for anyone embarking on a journey in the realm of sexuality.

Challenge Your Assumptions About Sex

𝓘 can't tell you the number of people who preface stories about their sexual experiences with "Well, I'm kinda freaky" or "My sex life is pretty boring" or "I'm not sure if this is normal." Trust me, no matter what you have or have not done sexually, there is someone else who has or has not done it, too. You can probably find a chat group online for those who like to wear diapers and chew Gummi Bears while someone sucks their earlobes. People's sexual experiences run the gamut from "I've never done anything, even with myself" to "Every day I do something with a feather duster." Human behavior around sexuality is unpredictable, diverse, and limitless. That's what makes it so wonderful. It's all normal . . . as long as it's consensual. But whether or not you're content with it is another story, and that's what this book is all about.

Basically, from the time we are born until the day of our death we are flooded with ideas about what is sexy and how sex should happen. In some ways the boundaries for sexuality are widening, but in some ways they are just as constrictive as ever. Every strong viewpoint that you have about sex is profoundly influenced by your past experiences and the messages you received. Often you're not even aware of how your experiences affect your interpretation of the world.

Where you are at this point in your life is the result of a lifetime of learning about sexual attitudes, values, and beliefs and your personal sexual encounters. Every sexual person experiences and expresses him- or herself differently. What you have learned and what you have done—combined with how our culture portrays sexuality—forms the basis for your "sexual script." This script generally specifies when, where, and with whom you have sex, as well as what you do sexually and why you tend to do it the way you do.

We are often limited by our own rules—we spend so much time worrying about doing things right, having the correct types of orgasms, being with a certain number of people, and how frequently to have sex that it's amazing we enjoy our experiences.

In her compelling and insightful book *Intimacy and Solitude,* Stephanie Dowrick says, "Many of us have sexual secrets about which we feel uneasy or even ashamed. These make us unusually vulnerable to real or imagined misunderstandings, attack, or potential ridicule." Once you realize that these "secrets" are normal, natural, and often common, you can start to accept them as a part of your sexual self and move forward.

One of the most compelling changes you can make is to challenge the assumptions that underlie your rules about sexuality. We all make them. And we are not immune to judging ourselves—often we are our own worst critics. We compare ourselves with others constantly (am I prettier, stronger, fitter, smarter, hotter?) and may have stringent rules about with whom, where, when, and how to have sex.

Examine Your Gender Expectations and Limitations

Gender expectations are a pretty tough thing to shake. Basically, we've been saddled with them since someone checked between our legs at birth and pronounced us to be a boy or a girl. Gender is a social construct, which means that you learn from family, community, and media how girls or boys should behave. The extent to which you ascribe to these roles (or not) can either limit or enhance your sexuality. For example, you may believe that if a woman asks for sex, she is a slut because you learned that a woman's role is to play hard to get and not "let" a man have his way with you too easily. Or maybe you are a man who doesn't have an enormous sex drive, but you learned that men are supposed to be perpetually horny and ready to penetrate anything, so you wonder what is wrong with you. Some of our most damaging and limiting assumptions are those we make about gender roles and sexual orientation.

Appreciate Your Body and Celebrate Its Sexual Capacity!

$\mathcal{P}$eople of all shapes and sizes have hot sex, and I guarantee that no matter how "attractive" the person may be, it is no indication of how hot the sex he (or she) is having will be. Sometimes the best-looking people have the worst sex. People who are comfortable with their bodies and their appearance often have better sexual experiences than those who are insecure. Getting to know your own body, whether through self-sexploration, learning the facts about how bodies work and respond, or having open conversations with others, is an important part of healthy sexuality.

Proceed at Your Own Pace

$\mathcal{T}$rying to change everything, to entirely re-create the sexual you all at once, is difficult, if not impossible. It's like the person who makes New Year's resolutions to go on a diet, exercise, cut down on drinking, and quit smoking all at once. By the third day, he or she is sore, hungry, and rummaging through the garbage can for old cigarette butts.

I remember reading one book that told me that in order to "spice up" my sex life, I should greet my partner at the door naked in nothing but Saran wrap, like a tasty dish waiting to be uncovered. All I could think about was that this would be the time Ed McMahon would ring my doorbell to tell me that I had won the Publishers Clearing House Sweepstakes and I would be on national television looking like a human fruit roll-up. While this may work for some, if you've never done anything remotely like it, it can be jarring for you and your partner. He or she may decide that you have truly lost it. And just because someone writes in some book that something is "hot" doesn't mean you're not if you don't want to do it. Trust your instincts.

Behavior change is best done incrementally. If you have never exercised, it would be irresponsible of me to encourage you to run a marathon the first day you get on a treadmill. It's the same with sex. If you are used to doing things in one particular way, I encourage you to introduce new ideas, positions, and products at a pace you find comfortable. Bottom line: Go at your own pace, challenge yourself but stay within your comfort zone, trust your instincts, and don't feel obligated to try everything.

Improve Your Communication Skills

*S*ex can be difficult and confusing to talk about. This is mainly because we don't learn how to talk about it. And many of us believe we shouldn't talk about it—that we should magically know what our partner wants and needs and that talking about sex ruins it. This astounds me. In what other aspects of our lives do we believe that *not* talking about something makes it better? Just imagine this scenario: "I had the best meeting ever at work. My boss didn't have to say a word. We sat down, he just looked at me in that special way, and I knew exactly what he wanted me to do; it was clear that I was supposed to do that report as a PowerPoint presentation." Usually people complain when they *haven't* been told what someone wants, when they have to second-guess what he or she wants them to do, or when his or her instructions are unclear—it is frustrating. Why doesn't the same hold true for talking about sexuality?

Expand and Enhance
Your Definition of Sexual Pleasure

𝒪h . . . Yes . . . Mmm . . . Ah . . . Ooo . . . Yummy. Sexual pleasures are unique, individual, and subjective experiences. You may never truly like porn or morning sex or keeping the lights on, and that is totally fine. What turns me on may turn you off. What leaves you trembling with desire may cause my vaginal juices to dry right up. Who cares?

Pleasure involves using your brain, harnessing your imagination, honing your five senses, trying new toys and techniques, and relishing physicality. Pleasure is one aspect of sexuality in which an animal comparison to birds and bees *does* make sense. In fact, animals are way ahead of humans in the sybaritic category, particularly in self-pleasuring (much to the embarrassment of many parents standing in front of the bonobo monkey cage at the zoo). Can you imagine mama monkey explaining to baby monkey that touching themselves is something to be ashamed of? The desire for pleasure is natural and normal.

The following quote from Paul Joannides's terrific book *Guide to Getting It On!* sums up what sex advice he would give if he were asked to limit his answer to one page:

> There isn't a feeling in the entire universe that you and your
> partner don't have stored, somewhere in your bodies, feelings
> that are waiting to be touched, shared and released. Yet the
> extent of your current lovemaking is to stick your tongues
> down each other's throats, tweak each other's nipples a
> perfunctory number of times, lick each other's genitals because
> that's what the sex books say you should do, and then thrust
> away until one of you goes "Ooo-ahh, Ooo-aah," and the
> other goes squirt, squirt, squirt. For a lot of people, sex is still

an extension of grabbing for the cookie jar, which is fine as long as your expectations aren't very high.

Fortunately, there are a lot of wonderful dimensions to sex besides just huffing and puffing while the bedsprings squeak. Sharing sex with a partner allows you to discover where the different emotions are stored in each other's bodies, where your hopes and dreams are hidden, where the laughter and pain reside, and what it takes to free the fun, passion and hidden kink. To achieve that level of sharing you have to take the time to know someone, to feel what they are feeling, to see the world through their eyes, and to let a partner discover who you are in ways that might leave you feeling vulnerable [author's note: even if your partner is you]. This can be scary.

Granted, there will be . . . times when all you want from sex is a quick jolt of sensation, but if that's all you ever expect from sex, then you might be coming up a bit short.

Be Prepared for All Contingencies

I once traveled to Europe with a friend who had irritable bowel syndrome. She forgot to pack her laxatives, and we spent an entire afternoon going to apothecaries trying to decipher how the homeopathic remedies offered for sale compared with Ex-Lax. Maybe you don't travel with the plethora of medical supplies that my brother, the doctor, does (antibiotic, anyone?), but you probably pack enough clean underwear and products for headache, upset stomach, and constipation, to name just a few. In other words, you take precautions, knowing that life involves risks. Sex involves risks, too, so being prepared with condoms and other safer-sex supplies goes with the territory.

Let the journey begin!

CHARACTERISTICS OF A SEXUALLY HEALTHY ADULT

(Adapted from SIECUS, *Life Behaviors of a Sexually Healthy Adult*, www.siecus.org/school/sex_ed/guidelines/guide0004.html)

What does it mean to be sexually healthy? According to SIECUS, a sexually healthy adult:

- appreciates his or her own body.
- expresses love and intimacy in appropriate ways.
- takes responsibility for his or her own behavior.
- enjoys sexual feelings without necessarily acting on them.
- seeks new information to enhance his or her sexuality.
- engages in relationships that are consensual, nonexploitative, honest, pleasurable, and protected against disease and unintended pregnancy.
- demonstrates respect for people with different sexual values and rejects stereotypes about the sexuality of diverse populations.
- assesses the impact of family, cultural, religious, media, and societal messages on his or her thoughts, feelings, values, and behaviors related to sexuality.

Chapter 2

HISTORICAL OVERVIEW

*Exploring the Messages
and Experiences You Got Around Sex*

* * *

Are you experienced?
—Jimi Hendrix

*Each of us is shaped by genetic/biological tendencies,
our general view of the world, our personality type, our level
of energy, our intelligence, the economic or social position of
our family of origin, the psychological health of that family,
the prevailing national and cultural norms, our religious
and social background, and so on.*
—Stephanie Dowrick, *Intimacy and Solitude*

The most appropriate place to start a sexploration is where most travel guidebooks start: with a historical overview—in this case, your sexual history. Not just a "first kiss/first intercourse/first wet dream" type of history, but a more complete, holistic view of the messages you got and the experiences you had that contributed to making you the sexual person you are today.

Where *did* you learn about sex? From your parents? Your woefully misinformed peers? The gym/health teacher at school? Nuns? An older brother or sister? How-to books? Movies? TV? Magazines?

What did you learn? What messages did you get about your body and sexuality? About sharing and loving? How did what you learned and the way in which you learned it affect your sexuality today?

Some of you may have had wonderful experiences and look back wistfully. Others may cringe or recoil when recollecting what happened in their lives, experiences shrouded in secrecy and shame, or the lack of information and preparation. Either way, memories are important stepping-stones in our journey and serve as barometers of how far we've come.

Our information about sexuality is a conglomeration of lessons gathered from people and events in all aspects of our life. We have had blatantly sexual messages and experiences as well as nonsexual lessons about being held and loved and about our bodies. Our parents or primary caregivers, our brothers, sisters, grandparents, and other relatives, peers and friends, intimate partners, religious leaders, school health teachers, and the media all deserve co-writing credit for our personal sexual scripts.

In the following sections, you will read people's stories about what influenced their sexuality. You'll also read examples in which no message was the most powerful message of all. Throughout the chapter are exercises that provide an opportunity for you to record your sexual memories and experiences: ones that had an impact on you, the stories you tell over and over, and the moments you question—really anything you want to write about and explore. You can start with messages you received when you were growing up, but also include more recent messages or things that others have said to you. Messages can be both verbal and nonverbal—often someone's behavior sends a message, too. The stories in the chapter will help spark your memories and give you examples of what others recall as relevant experiences.

At the end of each section, in the space provided, you'll be able to assess the impact of the messages you received and the experiences you had on your thoughts, feelings, values, and behaviors related to sexuality.

Remember, there is no right or wrong way to address this topic, only *your* way. Go where your mind leads you and try not to censor your responses. Whatever you recall has meaning to you, and that's important. Use the debriefing questions at the end of the chapter to help you think more specifically and comprehensively about what and how you learned and how it impacted on the sexual script you use today.

Your Origins

*Y*ou emerge from the womb all mushy, squooshy, and warm into the unpredictable world . . . of your family. Your immediate needs as an infant are simple at that point: to feel safe, secure, and loved. These remain basic needs for everyone. Our family of origin and our primary caretakers are the ones who can fulfill our basic, primary needs—or not. They are the ones who teach us about how we should interact with the others and how others should interact with us. They create the environment in which we learn key information about our sexuality and play crucial roles as we develop sexually.

Simon, thirty-six, was reared by a single mom until he was nine years old, and then he lived with his dad:

"Being in single-parent households where both parents dated was educational for me. My mom and dad had very different approaches. My mom was more sexual, and she had a lot of different guys coming around. They would hang out at the house, and she would kiss them and touch them in front of me. It made me uncomfortable, especially if

I had friends over, too. My dad, on the other hand, was very discreet about his dating. He would always tell me that he was going out with 'friends' when he was really going out with a date. I knew he was dating, and it made me feel that he was ashamed of me and that he didn't want any of the women he dated to meet me. I guess somewhere between my mom and my dad is normal, but I've always been confused about where I fit in."

Wendy, forty-two, remembers how her father would always come into her room without knocking on the door: *"I had no real privacy. Once when I asked him if he could please knock if the door was closed, he said that it was his house and what was I trying to hide. I wasn't trying to hide, I just wanted some privacy. So the next day I barged into his bedroom when the door was closed. There he was in all his naked glory. He put his hands over his crotch, ran into the bathroom, and yelled at me to get the hell out. I was stunned and I got punished, but he never came into my room without knocking again."*

Samantha, a fifty-three-year-old woman who has experimented sexually with both men and women, recalls how important her grandmother was to her appreciation of touch: *"My grandma was an incredibly sexy, sensual person. She lived with us, and we were very close. I remember being about five years old, sitting curled up in her lap and playing with her breasts, they were so fascinating to me. She pulled me close and whispered, 'Explore if you want, it's okay.' I felt safe and secure, and she helped me to feel good about my body and female sexuality."*

Dan, thirty-eight, says that his father was very hands-off when it came to touching or hugging: *"My father was an ear, nose, and throat doctor and spent his entire day literally in people's faces. When he came home at night he wanted to be as far away from people's faces as possible, including our faces. I don't remember hugging or cuddling with him, and when he kissed me it seemed perfunctory, as if it were an obligation. That was always my image of what a man should be, a bit standoffish and removed. I definitely absorbed those lessons."*

Sex Education, AKA "the Talk"

"When my father tried to have the 'sex talk' with me, it was the most awkward conversation ever," says Sean, twenty-seven years old. *"Part of me was laughing at his inability to say the word* penis *out loud without stuttering, and part of me was embarrassed at having to sit there and listen to what he was saying. I was fifteen at the time, and I'd already had sex. He was way too late with the talk, but I certainly wasn't going to tell him that."*

Mikel, forty years old, recalls the lame sex talk that his father gave him: *"I was about fifteen years old, and I didn't get anything out of it. My dad was a really good-looking guy, and before he was married, he went out with a lot of women. He seemed really confident, which I was not. I wish he would have taught me how to approach women and be more confident. That would have been more helpful than the sex stuff he tried to explain."*

Sharon, twenty-one, was fourteen when she started dating an eighteen-year-old and having sex: *"We used condoms, and I felt like I was being safe. My mother, whom I had not told about losing my virginity, stated that she wanted me to go on the pill. It caused a fight because I felt it was my decision to make and she shouldn't tell me to go on the pill. Then my mother shared her own story with me and told me that at fifteen she had sex for the first time, got pregnant, and had an abortion and that's why she wanted me to go on the pill. I decided I would go on the pill, and I felt so honored that my mother had shared that with me. And even though it was a young age to be sexually active, she was always supportive no matter what."*

"I grew up in the Bronx," explains Annette, fifty-four. *"One day my mother took me into the bathroom and closed the curtains. She gave me a tampon book called* Growing Up and Liking It. *She told me when a young girl gets a little older she developed hair on her private parts. I asked her where that was, and she just said, 'Down there,' so I was confused. And then I got scared because she told me that every month you will get your period, which means you can have a baby. She*

told me not to let boys touch me or I would have a baby, but she didn't explain anything else. It was horrible."

Kim, twenty, had this to say: "I'm an Asian, first of all, and typically many Asians are traditionally conservative and would rather die than risk embarrassing themselves over such a personal matter. Needless to say, I have the typical Asian parents, so yes, other than the fact that they told me not to lose my virginity until I was wedded, they didn't tell me anything."

"I first came across the word orgasm when I was twelve years old and secretly reading The Joy of Sex in my parents' bathroom, where they kept it (not so well) hidden," recalls Courtney, thirty-one. "Curious about what this word meant, I finally had an opportunity to ask my mother about it one day during one of our girl outings to the city. We got on the very noisy subway; I asked her, loudly, what an 'organism' was. Of course, as I was saying the word organism the train stopped in the tunnel and it got very quiet. My mom turned red and murmured that it was something adults did that felt good. The train started up, and she changed the topic. She never mentioned it again. I figured it was something that you didn't talk about. It wasn't until I was in college that I actually learned what it was."

"My mom told me that sleeping with someone before marriage is like using someone else's toothbrush," says Suzy, fifty-three. "She also couldn't eat shrimp with lobster sauce at a Chinese restaurant because she thought it looked like ejaculate."

ACTIVITY: WHAT I LEARNED ABOUT SEX FROM MY FAMILY

For each message that you recall, decide whether it reflects a positive, negative, or neutral attitude about sexuality. There are no right answers for this part; consider mainly your interpretation of the message. If you received no messages from your parents, for example, you may consider that negative because sex wasn't talked about.

What messages did you get from your family about sexuality? What was the sexual climate in your household?

_____

_____

_____

How did this impact on your sexuality?

_____

_____

_____

School

𝓜isinformed or knowledgeable, supportive or ostracizing, validating or intimidating, nasty or nice: Whatever messages you got about sex from your peers and from any formal sex ed that you had in school are bound to have influenced your later views in some way—or at least given you a moment's pause to wonder, "Now why did I sneer every time I saw Jessica Nichols in the halls? Oh yes, it was because we called her 'Chestica Nipples' and assumed she was a big slut because of her big breasts."

Rainy, twenty-nine, says, *"I grew up in Canada, and after talking to American friends, it sounds like we got pretty decent sex ed. We started in grade five, and I remember the teacher talking about masturbation and condoms and stuff like that. By high school we were a little more jaded and laughed at the sex ed we got, but we always had condom machines in the bathrooms and flyers for the free teen clinic in the counselor's office. Every girl I knew, knew where to get the morning-after pill by the time she was thirteen."*

This is a far cry from twenty-five-year-old Tim, who simply says, *"Sex ed? Nope, never had it."*

Huang, twenty, says, *"My school got funding for an abstinence only program. We learned that if we had sex we would probably die or ruin our lives. I remember someone asking, 'But what if someone has sex and doesn't want to have a baby, what should they do?' The teacher looked at the kid as if she were really disappointed and said, 'If you have sex, you have to face the consequences. But if you don't have sex, you have nothing to worry about.' What kind of answer is that? How hard would it have been to tell the kid where the condom aisle in the drugstore was? A few girls in my graduating class dropped out to have babies, and I wonder if that would have happened if they had had better information."*

Your Religious Upbringing and Your Sexuality

Whether you grew up Protestant, Catholic, Jewish, Buddhist, Muslim, Zoroastrian, Mormon, Hindu, Unitarian, Wiccan, or agnostic, you were probably indoctrinated with a belief system that specified with whom, under what circumstances, and in what manner you should engage in sexual activity. Although religious doctrine can get a bad rap when it comes to sex, it is best not to make sweeping generalizations and assume that all faiths conform to similar views on the subject of sexuality.

Naturally, a lot of the rules we learn are broken—frequently, that's part of growing up. The Catholic Church may say that sex is for procreation only, but many practicing Catholics use birth control. Similarly, you might have been taught that sex before marriage is a sin, but you and your girlfriend have a healthy sexual relationship and you don't see why that is a bad thing. You may have listened to sermons declaring, "Abortion is wrong," yet found yourself in the position of needing one. Maybe you grew up hearing that sex between two men or two women is forbidden but felt attraction to someone of the same sex. Many of the messages just listed promote sex as shameful and immoral, encouraging secrecy and silence about our sexual lives.

Contradictory beliefs and actions may result in guilt and shame that can have an impact on your sex life. Many people are able to reconcile their religious beliefs with their sexual selves by adhering selectively to religious practices they believe in and disregarding those that don't fit into their belief system. For others it isn't that easy.

Sunita, twenty-two, explains, *"If anyone thought I wasn't a virgin in my [Hindu] community, there would be no way I could ever get married. It's tough because my family moved here, sent me to American schools, let me wear American clothes, but when it comes to certain things still expects me to live like we are still in India. If they ever knew what I've done, they would disown me. Sometimes I feel all right about my choices and sometimes I feel terrible, like I have shamed my community."*

"The older I got, the harder it got to go to church," says Jamie, forty. *"I don't know exactly how old I was when I realized I was probably gay, but I do know that I would never be able to tell anyone. I heard too many sermons about what happened to people like me, and I was pretty much resolved to keep my feelings a secret forever. It caused me a lot of unnecessary stress."*

These stories reflect some typical assumptions about religion and sex and highlight the guilt and misinformation that are often associated with a religious view of sexuality. But there are those who received positive messages about sexuality from their religions.

Joe, thirty, remembers, *"The Unitarian Church that I went to was very serious about proactive sex education. They showed us filmstrips and slides that were frankly pretty pornographic. In a way, I don't know how they got away with it. We laughed and felt mildly uncomfortable, but I think that because of that I don't have the same type of religiously imposed guilt feelings about sex that a lot of other people I know do."*

Ella, twenty-nine, says, *"My experience with religion was mainly being sent to Jewish summer camp. Summer camp was coed and all about hooking up. In some ways I think that the idea was to make sure that Jews ended up with Jewish partners. So it really felt like as a teenager it was okay to experiment with sex, and that was part of the fun of being Jewish."*

For many people, a relationship with a religious tradition does not end when they leave home but is something that continues throughout their lives. Marta explains, *"As a Wiccan I view everything as being in harmony. This includes my sexuality. I truly feel that my relationship to the Goddess helps me channel sexual energy between myself and my partner and the earth, and because of that sex seems not only physically meaningfully, but spiritually fulfilling as well."*

Eitan, twenty-seven, a dedicated Jew, writes, *"My ethics and beliefs influence my every decision. Kindness towards others, truthfulness & appreciation, these are the tenets of my faith, and I try to bring them to all my relationships. How do religious ethics affect my sex life? I make sure every girl I sleep with has religious ethics!"*

Rashida, thirty-eight, explains, *"I appreciate that my religion gives me guidance about what is and is not acceptable in all aspects of life including sexuality. I think it would be so difficult to try to figure these things out without some sort of direction. I waited until marriage to have sex and didn't feel that it was a struggle at all. Actually it was much more of a relief to know that for me it just wasn't a choice."*

What messages did you get from your religion/religious leaders about sexuality?

_____

_____

How have these messages impacted your sexuality?

_____

_____

The Media

*O*ne of what Oprah calls "aha! moments" of sexual learning happened to me while I was watching the movie *Shampoo* (a Warren Beatty "sexcapade"). There was Warren on-screen, under the covers with Julie Christie, moving up and down and up and down and up and. . . . Well, you get the picture. Whoa. Revelation! People moved during sex. Who knew? Certainly not I; no one had ever explained to me how the mechanics of sex worked beyond the old sperm-meets-egg description. Few people I met over the course of my life were truly ready, willing, and able to discuss sexuality with me. So I learned a lot from the movies and books, and not surprisingly, I had a pretty unrealistic understanding of how it went down. I was not alone in my thinking.

Charlotte, thirty-seven, says, *"My mom did try to talk to me about sex, but most of my learning came from* The Sensuous Woman *and other books authored by people whose names were initials (by "O" or "J") that she kept in her bedside table. I would sneak them into the bathroom to read. There was this great exercise in one of the books. It involved eating an ice-cream cone in very specific ways, making intricate swirls with your tongue and teasing the peak with your lips. Not knowing why I needed such tongue technique, but eager to practice, I talked my parents into a trip to the local Dairy Queen. There I was, happily tonguing my vanilla soft-serve cone in the backseat of the car, when my younger brother looked quizzically in my direction. 'What are you doing?' he asked, catching me midswirl. My mom turned around and saw me lasciviously licking away. She didn't say a word, but the next time I looked in her bedside table, the books were gone. Lesson learned: Do not reveal what you know, and definitely do not practice in public or the books will disappear."*

Nina, thirty-six, recalls, *"When I was eleven and twelve, I used to cat-sit for the old lady who lived across the street. She lived alone and had tons of Harlequin romance novels and sexy Erica Jong–type books piled all over her house that I would sit down and leaf through. On the one hand I knew that they were nonsense, but on the other hand I was totally intrigued. I remember this one scene where a wealthy older heiress (she was probably supposed to be only thirty or so) had sex with the young pool boy and schooled him on technique, forbidding him from putting his entire penis inside her and teasing him with her vagina. I went home wondering how I could ever be sexy enough to actually tell a guy how to have sex with me."*

Chen, twenty-eight, explains, *"As an Asian American man, there were no images of sexy men who looked like me in the movies. There was only Bruce Lee, and he was just tough. I got the message that Asian men are not sexy, which was reinforced as I got older and my female friends all wanted to date Caucasian men."*

What messages did you get about sexuality from the media (such as television, movies, Internet, books, magazines)?

_____

_____

How did what you learned impact your sexuality?

_____

_____

REFLECTIONS ON WHAT YOU LEARNED

Review your answers to all of the "What I Learned" sections in this chapter before answering the following questions. These questions are written to help you reflect upon what you wrote and to glean understanding about your sexuality.

From whom did you receive the most messages? Were these mainly positive or negative?

_____

_____

What were the conflicting messages?

_____

_____

What messages did you get that were guilt or shame provoking?

_____

_____

What messages had the largest impact on you, and why do you think that is?

_____

_____

What messages did you get about women and sexuality?

_____

_____

What messages did you get about men and sexuality?

_____

_____

How did the messages you received influence your sexual self-perception?

_____

_____

What messages do you wish you had received about sex?

_____

_____

From whom would you have liked to receive those messages?

_____

_____

Other thoughts and reflections:

_____

_____

_____

Your Experiences

*W*hat were the key formative events and milestones on your sexual experience timeline? I've pulled out some of the general categories of experiences and some mainstream firsts below, but they may not reflect your life or what you would choose to highlight. Use them for inspiration and reflection, to spark other memories, or as pure entertainment.

First Show-and-Tell

"Playing doctor" is often our first experience with seeing and touching someone else's genitals. Role-playing starts early! Children have an innate and healthy sense of curiosity about their own and the bodies of other children, especially those that are different from their own. Here are a few thoughts from several people we spoke with:

"When I was about four and my sister was seven, she told me that she did not have a 'pee pee.' I asked her what she had, and she said she had a hole but nothing stuck out like mine. She agreed to let me see it, and I was so fascinated by what she said she peed from. We were checking out each other's genitals when Mom walked in on us and yelled at us." Chuck, thirty-four.

Chuck's recollection is pretty common. Even the smallest kids can tell the difference between men and women. Men have beards. Women have breasts. But most kids are baffled by differences they can't see and have to learn through furtive discovery:

"I grew up with two other sisters, and when I was eight years old I decided that it was time to see what a penis looked like. I knew I

couldn't ask my dad, so I asked my friend Thomas, who was my age and lived down the block. He agreed to show me his 'willy.' We went up to his bedroom, and he pulled down his pants and underwear and let me touch it. I touched it, and it started to get hard with a small erection. After I checked it out, we played a game of Battleship. The next week, Thomas came to my house and asked to see my 'down there.' We went into the bathroom, locked the door, and first I watched him pee. Then he asked if he could watch me. When I wiped myself he asked me to bend over so he could see between my legs. He looked very closely and said it looked cute. After that, we never talked about it and never did anything like it again." Linda, thirty-nine.

Linda's experience is also pretty typical but, unfortunately, the kind of activity that might get kids in trouble if they are caught. Parents are often at a loss for how to deal with the situation. In the film *Jersey Girl* (yes, the Jennifer Lopez–Ben Affleck post-breakup box office bomb), Affleck plays a single dad who walks in on his six-year-old daughter playing a game of "I'll show you mine if you show me yours." He is flustered and tries to have a conversation with his daughter and the little boy, but instead of schooling them on why what they did was wrong, he simply exposes his own embarrassment. This is a pretty typical reaction. Parents may feel instinctively that it is wrong for kids to explore but when pressed for reasons can seldom come up with anything cogent. As a rather angry father once said to my friend after finding her in her bedroom with a closed door and a boy, "It's just not seemly." Though the archaic language he used provided us with countless laughs for many years afterward, his point was a common one. It's viewed as not seemly to show someone else your genitals or to explore them unless it is under strictly prescribed circumstances—for example, heterosexual marriage. But I'll say it a million times until you are sick of hearing it: Genital exploration is natural and healthy.

"Playing doctor," becomes passé for many in their adolescent sexual exploration, at least for those in the following stories.

They've moved on to same-sex exploration in a "pretend that you're a boy or a girl and let's practice what it would be like" scenario:

"Before I had girlfriends, I had a best friend and we jerked off in front of each other, sometimes doing it to each other, and we had pretend sex, but never gay sex because we weren't gay. I think we just wanted to see what it felt like, but we didn't have girlfriends to try it out with." Robbie, thirty.

"I was thirteen and I wanted to show my best friend, Patti, how I played with myself. I actually began performing for her, and she got so turned on that she had to put her hands on me. She stroked my nipples and slipped her finger inside me. It was the most marvelous feeling I can remember." Cyndy, twenty-five.

"I was thirteen and sleeping over at my best friend's house. We were curious about boys, and we were always practicing dancing together so we would be prepared if one ever asked us to dance. That night we talked about making out and what we would do and not do. We started 'practicing' making out. We kissed and it was fun. Then we started French-kissing and really got into it. We went from there to rubbing our breasts. Then my friend suggested we take a shower. I think we were getting hot and didn't recognize it. Anyway, we got in a shower and soaped each other. We were still pretending it was a boy/girl. Having my breasts washed felt so good. I did the same for my girlfriend. She kind of leaned back into me as I soaped her breasts and pinched her nipples. Then I put my hands between her legs and felt her hair. I rubbed her lips, and she guided my hand to her clit. I touched her till she came. We then toweled off and got in bed. She got on top of me, and we kissed for a while. She sucked my tits, then went down on me. It was explosive." Jennifer, twenty-seven.

"When I was fourteen I wondered why all the boys would talk about pussy and cum and stuff, so I asked my friend what all this meant, and she told me it was too hard to explain, so she showed me. . . . My friend told me that she was going to put her finger in my vagina. I said, 'Okay,' and it felt really weird and tingly, and then she said, 'Now I'm going to rub your vagina.' That felt nice, too. When she put her tongue

inside my vagina, I think I fell off the bed. 'Does it feel good?' she asked. 'Yes,' I moaned." Serena, twenty-four.

What were your experiences with genital exploration? Did you play doctor with siblings or friends? Did your experiences involved same-sex exploration? Write about your experiences in the space below (use extra paper if necessary).

_____

_____

In what way did your experience impact on your adult sexuality?

_____

_____

First Kiss

Ah, the romance . . . the anticipation . . . the excitement . . . how time seems to slow down and the rest of the world disappears and the music plays and . . . Oh, I'm sorry, I'm actually recalling a "first kiss" scene from a movie. Truth is that my own first kiss story is not so romantic.

At the age of fifteen, I discovered (much to my distaste at the time) that "French"-kissing involved someone putting a tongue in my mouth—something my mother had told me was a sure-fire way to get germs. I was disgusted. When our faces awkwardly came together, this person suctioned onto my face, drooling saliva and probing the inside of my mouth with a flittering hummingbirdlike tongue. I couldn't wait to get back to my house. I must have brushed my teeth at least ten times and used an entire bottle of Listerine after that experience. Happily, in time and with better kissers, I overcame my aversion to

French-kissing and learned to enjoy it, particularly when I was kissing someone with whom I had chemistry—unlike that first person, forever deemed the "suction face kisser." But that's me.

Here's what others have to say about their first kiss:

"When I was eleven years old, I was going over to my boyfriend's house for the first time, but I was nervous about it. My friend said that I had to use Bonne Bell Lip Smackers so my lips would be nice and soft for kissing. Kissing?! I didn't know anything about kissing! I asked her whether I should keep my mouth open or closed; she said to keep my mouth closed. So, I get to his house and we're innocently playing Nerf basketball in his room when suddenly he pounced on me. What I re-member was that his kiss was very wet and slobbery, and it was open mouth. I didn't like it at all." Melanie, thirty-eight.

"The first boy I ever dated kissed with a soggy open mouth. Every time his mouth opened around mine, I felt as if I were being forced to lick the side of a stagnant well. His tongue was a live, wriggling fish that reeked of algae and muck that left a trail of glistening slime across my lips. Still, I never thought to stop kissing him. I was fourteen. I fig-ured everyone's mouth must taste like a cesspool, that even my own mouth was a gaseous, noxious thing. I figured that kissing was just an-other of those nasty things that adults had to endure, like scraping din-ner plates and wiping baby's asses. One thing I couldn't figure out was how kissing led to sex—all it made me want to do was brush my teeth.

"When my next boyfriend came along, I suggested other things, things that didn't involve our mouths so much: his hands across my ass, my fingers inside his shorts, his thigh between my legs. Eventually, of course, he wanted to kiss me. I was nervous but obliged. When he opened his mouth, I tasted the ocean, sea salt, and sunshine. I couldn't get enough of him, I wanted to suck out his tongue like a clam from a half-shell, I wanted to lick him dry and wait for the waves to wet him again. It was my first taste of true desire." Tiffany, twenty-nine.

"My first kiss took place at Hanna's house, at her twelfth birthday party. She suggested that we pair off and play that game where you go into the closet. Zev, Hanna's boyfriend, leaped up, grabbed her hand,

and pulled her into the laundry room. The door clicked shut. I looked at Betty, my girlfriend. I raised my eyebrows, like, 'So what do we do while we wait?' Betty threw me onto the couch, her palms slamming my shoulder blades down into the cushions. She wriggled on top of me. Our heads closed in. Her nose pressed into mine. My hands grabbed at air, my arms were trapped under her, immobilized. We squirmed against each other like restless gerbils in a cage. Our noses bumped. Betty grabbed my hands and said, 'This is not working.' She pulled me into a sitting position. She reached behind my head and pulled me in. I angled left, she angled right, and we connected. She tasted like candy and pizza and Diet Coke, all the foods that defined us. My brain exploded in blazing fireworks, and I felt as if my blood vessels were popping. 'Was this what having an orgasm was like?' I thought. Her tongue brushed mine. Our tongues could interact with each other! Wow.

"My eyes, which were closed, popped open for a second. I don't know if I heard something subconsciously, or I wanted to see myself kissing from the side, or if I just felt like a moron for having my eyes closed. But I opened them and there, in the unlit basement, stood Hanna's mother with a pink birthday cake in one hand and a cake knife in the other. She dropped the knife and it fell so that the blade stuck in the floor. We were all startled into silence." David, forty-five.

Describe your first kissing experience.

_____

_____

_____

How did this experience impact on your sexuality?

_____

_____

_____

The Big "V"

Ah, virginity. In our culture and in many religions, there is much stigma, ceremony, anticipation, and anxiety around doing the horizontal mambo for the first time. Sometimes it's described as something one person "gives" to the other, like a present (often the female). In other lingo, it's something that you "take," which implies a most unpleasant power dynamic. Most commonly it's described as something that you "lose"—a word choice that reflects a value that's put on "purity" as a positive and "sex" as a negative (particularly for women). When a boy has sex for the first time, he becomes a man, but a girl is no longer considered "pure." For some, virginity can become a "burden," something that you just are tired of being and want to get over. Some are proud of being virgins, and others are ashamed that they have yet to have "sex" (whether by choice or circumstance).

"Virginity" is one of those words without a universal definition, usually described in a heterosexist way (as in the penis enters the vagina). This is problematic, of course, for those who choose to have same-sex experiences or identify as lesbian or gay. At what point are they no longer virgins? Here's what several people have to say about virginity:

"I'm a lesbian, so losing my virginity didn't mean having someone put his penis in my vagina. Sexual intercourse, for me, is more difficult to define. For lesbians, sex is different things to different people—could be oral sex, penetration using digits, penetration using toys, etc." Caitlin, twenty-eight.

"The first time I had sex it was with this girl who was a friend of my brother's and she was two years older than me. I had masturbated before, so I knew what cum was, but when I was inside her and about to come, I didn't know what to do. Was I supposed to come inside her or get the hell out before I let loose? I was clueless, but since she didn't say anything like 'What the fuck are you doing?' I just kept going and came inside. We didn't use a condom, which was really stupid." Pierre, twenty-nine.

"The man I am seeing knows that I am a virgin. We started out as friends, and he teases me and we both laugh about it, and he reminds me that it most likely won't be as orgasmic as I hope. I know he likes the fact that I am a virgin, but he does have a hard time understanding why I have chosen to wait." Simone, thirty-three.

"I was the last one in my group of friends to lose my virginity. Most of them regretted losing it on drunken one-night stands and felt used and dirty afterwards and told me to make it special." Barbara, forty-one.

"I had been going out with a guy for a mere nine months and we had talked about making love, but I was nervous and so was he. We were both virgins. We got our hands on a series of videos that were very useful and full of information. On the night we made love for the first time, it was fantastic! It was just so natural. We had about thirty to fifty minutes of foreplay (maybe even longer) beforehand, and he performed oral sex on me, which made me orgasm. I gave him oral sex, although he stopped me before he 'came' in my mouth. It was the most enjoyable event in my life. There was no pain, no bleeding, just a night of pure sexual enjoyment. We ended up having intercourse a total of six times that night. We used condoms as our means of protection. He was and still is a fantastic lover—we are still together." Charlotte, thirty-five.

"The first time I had sex with a girl, I thought it was going to be really awesome. But it was actually really bad, and it hurt a lot. She tried to shove her hand into my pussy dry, and she was the worst person I have ever kissed. It was like kissing an overly aggressive teenage boy. She was really into antigentle sex. That can be okay sometimes, but this was just awful. I was so excited to be having sex with a girl that I was actually really into the experience, even though it didn't feel good. I had really wanted to be with a girl for a long time, and it was only later that I realized how bad the sex felt. I had sex with her two times, and I didn't come either time." Tamara, twenty-nine.

"I was seventeen years old. Well, it actually felt good to be close and to be so intimate with another person. It was almost like this weight was suddenly lifted from me. I felt I was the last girl on the planet to lose her virginity. I know that sounds crazy! I found out later that a few of my

girlfriends hadn't actually even had sex yet; I suppose girls lie about it, too." Svetlana, forty-four.

"It was a little uncomfortable at first, no blood, thank God, and he had no idea I was a virgin. He was gentle and loving, and I was very re-lieved that it felt so right. Problem number one came about six weeks later when I found out I was pregnant. I could not believe it! How the hell could this happen to me? I just was not ready for that. We used a condom, but obviously it didn't work for me. I am still with this person, happily married (well, sometimes). But it goes to show that if you think you are ready to have sex, it should be with a person you are in love with and have a relationship with, not just someone to sleep with. My daughter is now fifteen." Ashley, thirty-two.

"I'm sort of on the edge of being a virgin, I guess. The closest I've been to making love was almost four years ago. A man I was dating briefly penetrated me, but once I started bleeding we stopped. I blamed it on my period, because I was too embarrassed to tell him I'd never had sex before. Although I'm sure he had to know. I think that I was pretty stiff, because it did hurt so badly. I was twenty-five when my first sex-ual experience happened. I never intended to wait that long. This is why I decided to just go for it with this guy, even though we hadn't dated that long. I knew him before we had dated, he was a friend. So I figured it was as good a time as any. I just wanted it out of the way. I was tired of being a virgin." Sonia, twenty-nine.

"When I was fifteen I hooked up with a guy who was twenty-one. We were dry humping, and he was fingering me. I had heard somewhere about a girl who got drunk and couldn't remember if she had actually had sex with someone. I wasn't drunk, but I was not experienced, so af-ter we finished fooling around I was very nervous and asked him if we had sex and I hadn't noticed. Actually I said, 'Did we fuck?' He looked at me like I was crazy. It was totally degrading. Then he told everyone we knew. It was the most embarrassing thing ever." Angel, twenty-seven.

"It signified that I had become a man. I was twenty-two years old. Both my girlfriend and I were virgins, and we had been going out for

about five months. She took me into a park and, without warning, took my trousers and pants down and masturbated me. She was in total charge, which is something I've always liked. To this day she treats me like a young boy in bed, and I can't get enough of it. She wanted to make sure I waited, and for the next month she pulled my willy at every opportunity but told me that I could only see her naked when she gave me permission. The moment she did I was in awe of her beautiful body and lovely pussy. We went out together one afternoon, and she told me that she had decided to take my virginity and allow me to take hers that night. It was the most amazing night, because the act itself was so tender and meaningful. She is now my wife, who still turns me on after thirteen years of marriage and sixteen years of sex." Jake, thirty-eight.

"I was twenty-two years old. It was with a prostitute, and she didn't seem to care in the least that I was a virgin. She led me through it all— for example, 'Would you like me to suck you?' I didn't use a condom (pre-AIDS), and it felt warm, wet, and very, very good. I came in a minute or two because she was pumping me hard. I never told anyone except my best friend and my first fiancée. She was shocked and hurt that I had lost it with a prostitute (it was seven years before I met her!). My second fiancée—who is now my wife—wasn't bothered in the least." Theo, forty-nine.

"I was twenty-four when I lost my virginity, and it was nothing like how I had hoped or planned. My girlfriend and I had been apart for the summer, and she was cooler and less into me when she came back. Our first night together, she lay on the bed, pulled her pants down, and encouraged me to lie on top of her. I looked at her nakedness and the spread of hair around her legs and thought perhaps this might improve our relationship. I felt her hand move to my penis and guide it into her. I was unhappy doing this and decided I should take some form of precaution, so I got up to get a condom from my brother's room. I came back and put it on in front of her and climbed back on top. There was no foreplay, no arousal, and no real love. In fact, I wasn't even fully aroused. I did eventually come, but it wasn't the earth-shattering experience I expected.

Worse was after climaxing I withdrew, leaving the condom inside her. I think our night of 'passion' was really a good-bye kiss. She broke up with me the next week." Lawrence, thirty-six.

"I was in high school and was very attracted to this girl, who had the hots for me, but I was hesitant. By the third date I felt like we were supposed to have sex, but I was scared, and when the time came, I got sick to my stomach and threw up on her. It was so painful, and I felt so inadequate." Justin, thirty-nine.

Describe your first penetrative sexual experience.

_____

_____

_____

_____

_____

_____

How did this experience impact on your sexuality?

_____

_____

_____

_____

The Big O

For a lot of people, sexual pleasure culminates in orgasm. Sometimes orgasm comes as easy as pie, when and how we want it. For others, learning to orgasm is a process. But like other firsts, our earliest orgasms tend to be memorable experiences, as recounted by the following people:

"I was sixteen and had borrowed a rather dry sociology textbook from the library about teenagers and sex. I must've led rather a sheltered

life up to that point, as I didn't even know what an orgasm was. Lucky for me, there were instructions (sort of, if you read between the lines and improvised) to be found in the pages of the book. I lay for what seemed like hours and rubbed at the pink, still virgin place between my legs. For ages, nothing happened. (Perhaps I was doing it wrong. Memory doesn't recall my technique.) I persevered, and suddenly—out of the blue— wow! A climax of stunning, limb-weakening proportions. I do remember gasping in shock/delight and crawling across my lilac-carpeted bedroom floor. What a discovery! Of course, once I'd tried it, there was no stopping me, and frequent nocturnal fumblings and rubbings beneath the sheets soon ensued. But subsequent orgasms just didn't seem the same. I'll always remember my first 'come' as a true innocent aided by a borrowed sociology tome." Desiree, twenty-six.

"My first really heavy petting was with my friend Vicky. It started by taking a shower together to save time and hurry up, but when we bumped into each other with all of the soap and water, we both knew something was happening. Later on that night, we went upstairs to her room and undressed. The feeling of another female's skin and breasts upon your body is something to experience. We rubbed and fingered each other and definitely orgasmed. This was an ongoing summertime activity that went on into our junior year in high school." Lillian, fifty-one.

"I was twenty years old, in college and with my first real boyfriend. I couldn't have an orgasm during sex with him (I could if I masturbated), and I was convinced that there was something wrong with me. He was very supportive and helpful, but the more we focused on it, the more pressure I felt to come, which made me totally uptight. I went to the counseling center on campus to talk to someone about my problem. She was great and assured me that I was not abnormal, just inexperienced. She suggested that I read Lonnie Barbach's book, For Yourself. *He and I went to Disney World during our winter vacation, and there, in our room, on New Year's Eve, after a glass of champagne, with fireworks going off over Cinderella's Castle, we tried a new position that worked! The Magic Kingdom certainly was that for me!"* Roxanne, forty-six.

"I was seventeen years old when I got married, and I had no idea what sex was all about. After we were together for eight years, I told my husband that my body was ready to experience something new. I didn't know what that meant, really, but my body was craving a release. He was threatened by it; he said, 'One day you're acting innocent and the next you're acting all sexy.' The marriage didn't last. I'm Latina, and when we got divorced my next partner was black. He was an amazing lover, and he taught me that sex is more mental and emotional than physical. He focused on me, and it gave me confidence; he taught me about my body, and I had my first orgasm at twenty-six years old." Agatha, thirty-nine.

"The first time I had sex was when I was thirteen. My boyfriend was going down on me in my parents' basement, and I started to come. Not having any idea what was happening, I thought I was starting to pee! I was so embarrassed that I pushed him away. Well, that was my first mistake, because after that no matter what I did, I could not come again, whether I masturbated or had sex with a partner. And I was totally not into oral sex. It wasn't until I was nineteen that I actually had an orgasm again with a super-relaxed and attentive boyfriend who convinced me that he actually liked going down on me and enjoyed all the associated tastes and smell." Rhonda, forty.

"My first orgasms were actually kind of painful experiences. I discovered masturbation at twelve or thirteen and would do nothing else during my free time. Unfortunately, I had not discovered lube, let alone saliva, so the result was a very raw penis. I couldn't give it up, and I never wondered if I was doing something wrong. I just assumed that pain was the price you had to pay for getting to cum." Malcolm, eighteen.

Describe your first (if you have had one) and/or other memorable orgasms.

_____

_____

What stands out about this experience?

_____

_____

How did this experience impact on your sexuality?

_____

_____

Other Firsts

"The first time I gave someone a blow job, I was totally unprepared. I mean, I had a penis and knew what happened when I came, but the sensation of actually having someone come in my mouth was totally unexpected, and I kind of gagged a bit, more from surprise than anything else. The guy I was with was really nice about it, but I was still embarrassed—especially because I hadn't told him it was my first time." Simon, twenty-one.

"I remember the first time someone went down on me. I couldn't feel a thing. I think the guy was so nervous that he was just too gentle. I was waiting for bells and whistles, and what I got was more like a whimpers and whispers. For a long time I just thought oral sex was kind of boring." Gwen, thirty-three.

"I was a late bloomer and very sexually inexperienced for most of my adolescence. When I was a junior in high school, I had my first boyfriend, and I was always afraid to be alone with him because I was fearful of any kind of sexual activity. One day, we were alone at his house after school and we were kissing. I started to feel all these weird sensations in my groin area and didn't know what to do. I went to the bathroom and my underwear was all wet. I thought there was something wrong with me, so I made up some excuse about having to go home. I broke up with him shortly after. No one had ever told me that my body would react to getting sexually excited and that it was normal to be 'wet' because of that. I feel sorry for myself that I was so uninformed and scared." Michelle, forty-four.

"*I was hooking up with a girl for the first time. We agreed not to have sex and just to masturbate together. She was lying on her back, and I was straddling her knees. I got really turned on watching her touch herself and got really into the moment, so I ripped off my shirt and started whipping it around in the air like a lasso. When she saw me doing this, she burst out laughing and I fell off her. It kind of killed the moment.*"
Jordan, twenty-nine.

"*I grew up learning that the anus was dirty—it had one purpose and one purpose only. The first time and last time someone tried to give me a rim job, I was mortified and could not believe that anyone would want to put their mouth there. I have friends who love giving and receiving that, but I just can't get over thinking about what goes on in the bathroom.*" Lisette, forty-one.

Life Changes

*S*tuff happens, and sometimes your life takes unexpected turns that can have a lasting effect on your physical and emotional capabilities. No matter how slight or severe, sad or painful, or ultimately positive and joyful, these changes can often affect your sex life:

"*I was in a really bad car accident a few years ago that really changed my life. I used to snowboard and mountain-bike, and now I just can't do that anymore. I have to take a lot of pain meds, which can make me kind of numb. So between the meds and the pain, sex can be tough. At first I was really depressed and would get so mad when people told me how 'lucky' I was to be alive. I didn't feel lucky, I felt like a crippled old lady. My boyfriend at the time couldn't really deal with it and we broke up, but I have a new boyfriend now. I don't think I would have dated him before—he's kind of overweight and not my 'type,' but if anything good came out of this accident, it is him. He is so respectful of my limitations that I have learned how to have sex again. He is really great about respecting that I can't have sex every day and that some positions are out of the question, but he also has made me realize that a lot of sex is still possible. He helped me have sex again, and I helped him quit smoking! Pretty good trade-off."* Erin, thirty.

"I went on antidepressants after years of resisting taking them because I was sure that being depressed was some human failing of mine. I was ashamed of my inability to conquer it, and I developed a perky, together persona to cover up the depression. But each day it was such a struggle to just get out of bed, and it took an enormous amount of energy to be functional. Finally, I started taking Zoloft. Within a month, I felt as though a gray fog had been lifted from around my head, and I knew that this was what I had needed. The side effect from the medication, however, is that it is much more difficult for me to orgasm. So now what I find myself doing is avoiding having orgasm in my sexual encounters. I take care of the man first and hope he'll fall asleep before it's my turn. Or I tell him that I don't know him well enough to 'let go.' I've even considered faking it, something I have never done. It's as though I think that I have to have an orgasm within a prescribed amount of time or someone is going to reject me if I tell him I'm on medication, or get bored if I take too long, so if I can't do that, I just give up. I've accepted my need to take medication but still judge myself about the side effects." Kelly, thirty-four.

"After my hysterectomy, my sex life was more unbelievable. Maybe it's because I don't have to worry about getting pregnant." Solange, forty-three.

"I have MS [multiple sclerosis], and I met this guy I was going to have sex with, but he told me he had herpes and I just freaked out. I couldn't imagine having another part of my body affected by something. As it is, I already feel really limited. I just can't deal with anything else that will make it harder to have sex." Dex, thirty-six.

A disability or illness is not the only thing that can change your body and affect your sex life. Pregnancy is something that impacts women's sexuality, whether or not they talk about it. Some women claim that they never felt sexier than when they were pregnant. Others remember feeling like an enormous blimp and that sex was the furthest thing from their mind. Here are some personal recollections:

"When I saw the heading entitled Sex During Pregnancy, I laughed out loud. Does this exist? If so—do women have to pay a male gigolo for an hour session? This is my personal experience: Sex During Pregnancy—Or Lack Of.

"Almost immediately after finding out that this wonderful accident had happened to us, our undercover antics took a complete nosedive and of the very nonsexual nature. Mother Nature is a funny thing, isn't she? I mean, when I first found out I was pregnant, I was shocked and the idea of sex was totally offputting on my part, mainly in case I caused any damage and the baby fell out (did I forget to mention irrational thoughts caused by raging hormones?), and my partner was rebuffed on many of his requests. Then, as your confidence in pregnancy grows, your waistline and sex drive do the same.

"Ironically, at that point your partner starts to recognize that there is now a third party involved in your sexual encounter and she is not a six-foot blond stunner! His previously persistent pestering dwindles to a faint whispered request for oral sex 'as long as you keep your neck down, hidden under the covers'! At this suggestion, you totally hate your partner and start to become more reliant on your battery-operated friend, sleeping in a separate bed (why should I give if I do not receive?). Anyway, my orgasm rate has never been higher—100 percent hit." Rosa, forty-one.

"As my due date approaches, I am starting to look forward to having rampant sex again—although I think this break has actually built up the sexual tension that seems to come when you're with someone for five years—however, technically I am almost a born-again virgin, so I'm looking forward to losing it for the second time—in between changing nappies, obviously." Tracie, thirty-five.

"I'm pregnant with my first child, and although I have a lot of physical discomfort, I have this amazing ability for multiple orgasms. My obstetrician told me that I should massage my perineum to make it less *likely to rip during birth, and my husband thinks that it's the greatest thing ever. It doesn't really turn me on, but he's having a great time between that and the multiple orgasms. We installed a massaging showerhead, and I use it every day to masturbate, which makes the pregnancy pains go away."* Jeanie, thirty-two.

A woman's pregnancy can affect her partner's sexuality, too:

"My wife was overdue, and her doctor told us that having sex would help bring on labor. 'Cool,' I thought. We laughed a lot trying to find a position that worked. When we finally figured it out and were doing the deed, I swear that I could feel the baby's head against the tip of my dick. That really freaked me out. I was afraid that I was going to hurt her or that she'd have some weird memory of something poking her in the head right before she was born. I just had to stop." Matthew, forty-three.

That said, pregnant women can, and often do, have tremendous sex appeal:

"Recently I went out with my friend Nina, who just had her first baby. Nina was the sexiest pregnant women I had ever met. She was out at every party in a tiny little dress exposing her ever growing belly and great cleavage. On the weekends I would see her lounging at the park in a bikini wearing huge oversize sunglasses and sporting a huge oversize belly. I heard more than one man remark, 'I never thought pregnancy was hot before, but damn! Nina makes it look so good.' And they were right, she did! So all you pregnant gals out there, remember, there's probably a little Nina in us all. No need to let a potential baby spoil your fun while waiting for the happy day to arrive." Emilia, thirty-two.

Describe a life-changing experience that had an impact on your sexuality (such as menopause, aging, disability, illness, or pregnancy).

———————————————————————

———————————————————————

———————————————————————

How did this experience impact your sexuality? Would you consider the impact of this experience to be positive or negative, or are you unsure?

_____

_____

_____

What were the commonalities among the experiences that you chose to write about?

_____

_____

_____

What surprised you about your experiences?

_____

_____

_____

What do your experiences tell you about the nature of your attraction to others?

_____

_____

_____

What do your experiences tell you about your comfort around being a sexual person?

_____

_____

_____

Were your experiences more positive or negative? Why do you think this might be?

_____

_____

What experiences had the largest impact on you, and why?

_____

_____

REFLECTION: PUTTING IT ALL TOGETHER

How do you think the messages that you got about sexuality (recorded in the first part of the chapter) are related to the experiences that you have written about in the second part of the chapter?

_____

_____

What theme or themes seem to emerge repeatedly for you?

_____

_____

_____

_____

Does recalling these memories make you happy? sad? nostalgic? make you laugh? shudder with embarrassment and regret? Try to explain why you think these feelings arise.

_____

_____

_____

_____

What are your rules around sexuality? Where did they come from? How do they affect your sexuality?

_____

_____

_____

How have your past experiences influenced how you feel about your body?

_____

_____

_____

_____

_____

How do you feel, in general, about the partners you have had?

_____

_____

_____

_____

_____

What did you think of the stories you have read? Do any stand out for you? Why?

_____

_____

_____

_____

_____

Chapter 3

PLANNING YOUR ITINERARY

Getting to Where You Want to Be

* * *

Our love and sex lives are only as mature as we are and not
more so—therefore mistakes and betrayals must happen.
—Damaris Parker-Rhodes,
The Way Out Is the Way In

*S*o, is your head swimming with all of the messages, experiences, and knowledge that the previous chapters evoked? What happens next? How do you make sense of what you've learned?

In Hollywood, when the story for a movie doesn't gel and the writers are struggling with the script, the producers bring in a "script doctor" to do rewrites and make it all better. The script doctor looks at the "big picture" and sees what needs fixing. He or she still needs to work with the actors who have been hired and the basic premise of the story and the scenes that have already been filmed—in much the same way that, in order for you to doctor your own sexual script, you must work with and respect your past, your physical ability, your emotional capacity, and your partner (if you have one), who has his or her own abilities. You can work to improve these things by learning new techniques, enhancing your emotional connections, and accepting your limitations. In this chapter, you serve as your own script doctor by deciding where and how your sexual script needs rewriting.

Hopefully, you have gained some insight into your own sexuality by doing the worksheets in the previous chapters. You may have realized how you view your own sexuality, why and in what way you prevent yourself from being a more sexual person, how you feel about sex, what messages and experiences helped you form those feelings, or even why it is more difficult to participate in certain sexual activities than others. You may have read some of the stories and have been repulsed by what was described. Or maybe your interest was piqued. You may be startled or soothed or disappointed by what you have learned about yourself. Some of you may be champing at the bit, ready to let loose on some new *sexcellent* adventures. As with any journey, the first step is to decide your destination.

In the space below or on a separate piece of paper, describe your current sexual script; for example, what you do or don't do, a typical sexual encounter—it doesn't matter if it's with someone current or in your past, with yourself, or in a fantasy.

_____

_____

_____

_____

_____

_____

_____

Go back to the section above and highlight what works for you in this description. What do you like? What feels good? What do you want more of? List these below.

_____

_____

_____

Now, go through the same section again and highlight what is *not* working for you, or what is dissatisfying for you, or where you feel least secure or judge yourself. List those things below.

_____

_____

_____

In the space below or on another piece of paper, write a paragraph describing what an *ideal* sexual encounter would look like for you. This can be based on a dream or fantasy, something in the previous chapters that piqued your interest, or an actual experience. Don't censor yourself, but instead write freely whatever comes to mind without analyzing or judging yourself.

_____

_____

_____

_____

_____

Now, underline or highlight what stands out for you in the lines above. What are the key elements in this scenario? Where does it take place? Who is your partner(s)? What are the activities that you are doing? Is anything about what you wrote surprising to you?

_____

_____

_____

How is this description different from your current sexual script?

_____

_____

_____

What Is Great Sex, and How Can I Have It?

*N*ow, where did I put that instruction sheet? Oh, here it is. Okay, insert part A into opening B and—violà!—you've got great sex. Ha! If only it were that simple. Truth is, sometimes it flows naturally and sometimes it's like trying to put together furniture from IKEA using only the Swedish directions.

Forty-year-old Margaret says, "*I feel like there are all these women out there doing things with ice cubes that I never got the hang of and so my partners are missing out on something.*" Well, Margaret and plenty of other folks might want to know that it's not that they have been left out of some supersexy secrets. There is only so much you can do with body orifices. The real secret of sexual exploration is not mastering the "frog position," it's about learning to understand and accept your needs, limitations, and desires— in other words, being okay with your sexual self. Coming to terms with unrealistic expectations about sexual relationships (for example, that they alone will fulfill you) and realizing that the messages we get from the media are often just idealistic images that humans cannot uphold can make us a lot better in bed than learning how to artfully dribble chocolate sauce onto someone's vulva.

Here's what some experts have to say in response to the question "What is good sex?" You may be surprised by some of their answers:

Whoever you're with, one of the keys to good sex, along with communication, is to know what you're into, but also keep an open mind. Countless times, I've thought that I knew exactly what cues my mind and body responded to, only to find them completely turned on their head. Just when I was convinced that I was a total bottom when it came to BDSM [bondage, domination, sadomasochism], I found that actually I can get just as turned on being a top. For me, so much of it depends on who it is I'm having sex with. Not that I change myself or my desires based on them, but that my desires themselves often change. I can sometimes get into a certain action, fetish, or position because someone I'm desperately attracted to is into it; if the person is special enough, sometimes it feels like anything they do can make the sex "good." For me, being fully present in a sexual encounter—by dropping my everyday cares and worries and committing myself to the enjoyment of the moment, to stating what I want and also listening to what the other person wants—goes a long way toward making sex the pleasurable escape it can be. When my mind is preoccupied, my body knows it, and I have trouble getting off. So even though it may seem slightly contradictory, knowing what you want, knowing what turns you on, what your limits as well as your needs are, is incredibly important. You might like someone but be able to tell on the first date that sexually you probably aren't compatible. On the other hand, your body just may surprise you, may sneak up and change things around when you least expect it, offering you new ways of getting off, so don't always rule something out simply because you think you might not like it. There is no magic formula for good sex, and everyone is different. You might want to do it twenty-four hours a day, while for someone else once a week might suffice, and you may very well encompass all sorts of differing sexual desires over your lifetime. The less time you spend worrying about "Am I normal?" and the more time you spend looking at "How can I get what I want sexually?" from yourself and your lover(s), the better your sex will be. Don't be afraid to test things out and experiment, whether it's with partners, porn, positions, toys, what have you.

—Rachel Kramer Bussel, editor, *Naughty Spanking Stories from
A to Z* (Pretty Dirty Things, 2004)

I really think what makes sex good is being able to laugh—about sex, during sex, after sex. We all have these images in our heads about steamy, intense passion where clothes slip away and we're carried away by lust. Afterwards we're draped in lovely sheets with every hair intact. The reality is far more funny—our bodies wiggle and jiggle, we make odd noises, zippers stick or we leave our socks on, makeup gets smeared, and sometimes body parts don't work the way we want them to. Afterwards, we're hot, sweaty, and look as if we've had a workout. That is when you can look at this person and just laugh because sex should be joyful. We should laugh because we're happy that our bodies have such a capacity for pleasure. We should laugh with this person and feel connected enough not to take the whole thing so seriously.

—Francesca M. Maresca, MA,
coordinator of health promotion,
Rutgers, the State University of New Jersey

The best sex and the most satisfying sex are not the same. I have had great sex with . . . intimate terrorists . . . who seduce and attract by giving you just what you feel your heart needs, then gradually or abruptly withholding it once they have gained your trust. And I have been deeply sexually fulfilled in bonds with loving partners who have had less skill and know-how.

—bell hooks, *all about love*

There are a bazillion books and videos about sexual techniques, and if they worked, people would be having a lot more fun than they seem to be having . . . it's about whether [you] can be absolutely present in a relationship. People always want to know that one trick that will drive their partner wild.

Most sex guides concentrate on "technique"—this position, that stroke, those toys. . . . Think back on your sexual history and replay in your mind one of your favorite sexual experiences. What were the key elements of this experience that made it so good for you? I'm actually willing to bet that the key elements didn't have much to do with technique at all and had more to do with passion and energy.

—Ann Marti, sexuality counselor, from *Thoughts on Pleasure,* Society for Human Sexuality (www.sexuality.org)

Here's how some nonprofessionals answered the same question:

"A good sexual experience for me is something that means something. As vague as this is, I mean that it is with someone whom I care about, whom I want to make happy, and who makes me happy. I don't need an orgasm for something to be a good sexual experience. I need to be happy. I like my neck, my ears, my lips, and my genitals to be touched. I like it when those parts are licked and sucked on or brushed with a simple finger or breath. I will not toss someone's salad or have mine tossed. That to me is nasty. I want to kiss someone when I am engaging in intimate acts with them, and after they do that, I cannot even think about it." Greg, twenty-four.

"My ideal sexual experience is to be with someone I love and who loves me. I definitely need to have a mental connection with someone to have a good physical experience. Someone's eyes, their chest, and their ass are also important in terms of what my first focus is." Nicholas, twenty-seven.

"Good sex is when you are with a guy who loves making love to

women and who is up for an entire hard-core session, not just having an orgasm and then it's over." Aimee, thirty-two.

"What makes for good sex? Trust, stamina, big cocks, losing myself in the experience, getting up and dancing, music, candles." Suzy, fifty-three.

"A good sexual experience means being with someone who allows me to be me, warts and all, and allows me to be afraid without judging me." Justin, thirty-nine.

What do you notice about these statements? I notice that for all of these people, good sex isn't about expert technique or mind-boggling orgasms, but more about relationships, connection, and feeling good about what they are doing.

Think back on your sexual history and replay in your mind one of your favorite sexual experiences. What made this experience so good for you?

_____
_____
_____

Now, reread both your real and the ideal scenario you wrote before. Based on what you wrote and your recollection of one of your favorite experiences, how do you define "good sex"?

_____
_____
_____

How is your definition of good sex different from or similar to the expert descriptions above?

_____
_____
_____

What part or parts of your ideal scenario can you imagine yourself actually doing?

_____

_____

_____

What would you need to know, do, or think in order to see yourself having your ideal sexual encounter?

_____

_____

_____

Bringing It Home

As with any journey, there is no way you will be able to explore all parts of a country in one trip. Most travelers pick one area or region to focus on. That's what I recommend for your sexploration.

The length of the process and the path that you take are determined by your comfort level. During your journey, you are developing not only new tastes, but a new language in which to talk about these tastes. You may never truly like porn or morning sex or keeping the lights on, and that is totally fine. Who cares? The goal is not perfection . . . you don't need to be the sex god or goddess of the world, just of your world. Bottom line: Go at your own pace, challenge yourself, but stay within your comfort zone, trust your instincts, and don't feel obligated to try everything. In some cases it's not only you, but your partner who is going on this adventure with you. He or she will probably have his or her own issues.

A lot of people come into sexual situations with preconceived notions about what sex should be like. Once we can shake these notions and acknowledge that not every sexual encounter should end in a series of mind-blowing multiple orgasms and leave you in a tangled mass of sweaty limbs, then we can move forward and work on our sexuality.

Dr. Betty Dodson, in her presentation during the Orgasm—Recent Models and Methods symposium at the 1998 joint conference of the Society for the Scientific Study of Sexuality and the American Association of Sexual Educators, Counselors and Therapists, describes one couple's experience:

> There was an older couple I worked with. She was in her early seventies and her husband was in his late sixties. She had never had an orgasm until I showed her how to use the electric massager. Since she felt masturbation was something that was private, she didn't feel comfortable doing it in front of her husband, so she'd go into the bedroom and use the massager alone. Meanwhile, he would be sitting in the living room kind of rubbing his dick, getting turned on listening to the old vibrator buzzing. When she'd call out his name, he'd jump up, run into the bedroom with a hard-on, get on top, and they would fuck. After having one orgasm masturbating, she could usually have another one with him. They were thrilled with this new arrangement. So who's to say how we have sex?

When sexuality counselor Ann Marti was asked to define the single most valuable insight a person can have that will improve that person's experience of relationships and sex, she replied, "People are not going to be very excited about this, but I think the commitment to your own personal growing up is what is going to give you a better relationship and sex life. . . . Clearing up your emotional garbage, whether that's through individual therapy or group therapy, is also helpful; we've all got it, and I don't know too many people who don't need a little bit of work getting through it so that when they come into a relationship they're not bringing Mom and Dad and every lover they've ever had to you."

She added, "Just because you're having functional sex doesn't mean you're having good sex; functional sex from a clinical standpoint just means you can have an orgasm. . . . Men, for example, can have an incredibly erotic sexual connection and the best orgasm of their life and never have an erection."

Here are just a few ways to make a change that you might not even have thought about; there are many more in the following chapters:

- Expand your definition of sex. Liberate yourself from the bonds of penetration-orgasm-equal-sex definition. Spend a night just kissing passionately and leaving your clothes on and label that sex. Take an afternoon to give your partner a back rub and call it sex. Truth be told, "goal-oriented sex" is less fun and more fraught with anxiety, which, since sex is how adults play with each other, takes all the fun out of it.
- Understand and appreciate how your body works.
- Challenge the assumptions you make about how, when, with whom, in what way, and where you engage in sexual encounters. Play with dominating and submissive roles, try new positions and activities, employ the power of fantasy.
- Improve your ability to talk about what you want, need, and expect for yourself and from others in your sexual relationships. Figure out what language to use, learn to "talk dirty," or try out new phrases.
- Explore the myriad ways you can give and receive pleasure. Enhance your sensory exploits.

When asked why they might want to undertake a sexploration, a few honest souls gave these responses:

"I want to be with someone who would allow me to be me—warts and all; allow me to be afraid and not have expectations that because I'm a man I don't have any fears around sex."

"I wish that my husband and I had sex more frequently. We have it about once a month, and I always have to initiate it."

"I have never had an orgasm."

"I want my partner to be more aggressive."

"I wish I enjoyed oral sex more."

"I want to feel more connected to my partner."

"I need to know my body better."

"I've had some bad experiences, and I haven't been able to enjoy sex in the same way since it happened."

"I have a bunch of fantasies that I want to try out with a partner, but I don't really know how to bring up the issue."

So here are some ways to start mapping out your journey to the land of good sex.

List what parts of your ideal scenario really get you going. What parts indicate great sex to you?

_____

_____

_____

Which of those are you not doing?

_____

_____

_____

Why not?

_____

_____

_____

What might you need to know, do, or think about in order to do this one thing?

_____

_____

_____

Now, what are the steps to getting there? Break it down. For example, if you want to role-play a massage therapist fantasy, you would need to

- read about massage.
- research lubricants and various massage techniques.
- figure out how to bring it up with your partner.
- buy the equipment and supplies.

Pull out one or two goals for your sexploration and write them below.

_____

_____

_____

_____

_____

Chapter 4

CULTURAL CONSIDERATIONS

Challenging Your Assumptions

✳ ✳ ✳

Sexuality here in America remains a confusing entity.
A "just say no" mentality thrives in a culture that uses
sex to advertise and sell everything from soap to beer.
As a result, there are times when we flaunt our sexuality
and other times when we deny it completely.
—Paul Joannides, *Guide to Getting It On!*

So you're ready to throw off society- and self-imposed shackles and make some serious changes. But something still seems to be stopping you. Hmm, now what could it be? Oh wait, I know! The rules! Most of your "rules" about life, such as where and when to vacation, whether or not to wear white clothes before Memorial Day weekend, and with whom and how often to have sex, are influenced by what you've observed and absorbed throughout your life.

Contrary to the adage, we *do* judge books by their covers. We make assumptions about others by the way they chew their food, wear boxers or briefs, the size of their breasts, or how they behave sexually. There seems to be some safety we derive from labeling people, placing them into specific defined categories (you are straight, you are gay), and expecting them to behave in a prescribed manner.

But people are more complicated than that. Just because a man has sex with a woman doesn't make him straight. Stereotypes about how you should behave because you are male or female, young or old, straight or gay, may have limited your sexual script in the past. But remember, identity is fluid, and being flexible about your role in sexual relationships is fundamental to your personal and sexual health.

What Is Normal?

We compare ourselves with others constantly (am I nicer? better looking? stronger? fitter? smarter? hotter?). We watch TV shows about make-overs as the way to happiness. We are bombarded with ideas that tell us the "right" way to eat, dress, smell, date, and look.

Rules can be sexually limiting—especially when we worry about doing things right, having the correct types of orgasms, being with a certain number of people, having sex a certain number of times each week.

This idea that there is some universal normal sexual barometer is a difficult notion to undo for many people. "Is it normal to . . ." is the most frequent beginning to the questions I am asked. People wonder about the shape, size, smell, and taste of their breasts, penis, vulva, or other genitalia (What is the normal penis size? Do most women have discharges from their vaginas?). They wonder about what they like to do or not do sexually (Is it normal to masturbate every day? Do other women like it when their partners put a finger in their anus? Am I a pervert if I like to videotape my sexual exploits?). They wonder about

> *Every culture has its own definition of what is sexually acceptable, erotic, and forbidden. The following examples from* Guide to Getting It On! *will give you a smidgen of the vast array of cultural difference:*
>
> • During the Summer Olympics, male gymnasts from the Russian team often celebrated good performances by kissing other team members on the lips. U.S. gymnasts wouldn't be caught dead doing that in public.
> • In Japan, it is common practice for people to strip naked and bathe together. Nobody finds this kind of public nudity to be erotic or shameful, but it's not okay for them to kiss in public. In the United States it's nearly the opposite: Kissing is fine (although the "get a room" heckling usually accompanies prolonged public displays of affection), but public nudity is a legal offense.
> • Women in Muslim cultures cover themselves from head to toe when appearing in public. Women in Hollywood appear in public wearing a few molecules of black spandex, designed more to expose than to cover. Who is the sexual prisoner?

the sounds and physical reactions that accompany their sexual experiences (Do other women cry when they have orgasms? Why do I fall asleep after I come?). They are concerned about their motives for choosing sexual partners (Is it bad to be a player? I just want to fool around now, not be with someone that I'd settle down with; am I a slut? I'm at a point in my life where I just want a hugging and kissing companion, not someone to have sex with; am I selling myself short?). One of the most compelling changes you can make is to challenge the assumptions of what is "normal."

What rules do you have about "normal" sexuality that are associated with your cultural background?

_____

_____

What are the assumptions that underlie these rules?

_____

_____

Some of the most ingrained rules are those we have about *gender roles*. At birth, gender is determined by checking between the baby's legs to see if it has a penis or a vulva. From that time forward, you are labeled male or female. Gender is how we are viewed in the world by society. Males and females usually have different expectations about how to dress, where to work, what activities to enjoy, and how they are supposed to interact with members of the same and opposite sex. *Gender bias,* which means holding stereotyped opinions about people according to their gender, can negatively affect your sexual interactions. Gender bias might include believing that women are less sexual than men or that men want only to have sex, not to connect emotionally. Unfortunately, we live in a world that judges women for having multiple sex partners and sex outside of a "committed" relationship. On the other hand, men who have multiple sex partners are often regarded as studs or players. These ideas can have lots of negative results. Women may feel ashamed or guilty about having sex, which can thwart healthy sexual development. They may downplay the number of sexual partners they've had. As a counterpoint, men may overreport the number of sexual partners they've had because of the expectation that they are supposed to be unbridled, perpetually horny sex machines. Not all men are that way—most are not even close—and that's a good thing. The pressure to perform is an enormous burden on the male of our species. A willingness to challenge gender role stereotypes can often help you break out sexually.

Most people's sex matches their *gender identity*. This means that if you have a penis, you feel male, and if you have a vulva, you feel female. Sometimes a person's sex and gender identity do not match or are discordant. This could be for a couple of reasons: Someone has an intersex condition, or someone identifies as transgender. Unlike intersex individuals, people who are transgender do not have physical conditions that cause gender discordance. For psychological and emotional reasons, their gender identities do not match their physical bodies. Transgender people with penises may identify as female, and vice versa. Many transgender people simply buck the system and do not identify fully as either male or female.

Gender Roles

𝒫ersonally, I don't like wearing stiletto heels, ruffled shirts, or pencil skirts. I love funky socks with stripes, vests, and chunky, clunky Doc Martens shoes. I rarely wear makeup, but when I do I whip out my M.A.C. cosmetic case filled with shadows, shiny lip gloss, and waterproof mascara. My favorite possession is my power drill (insert sexual innuendo here!), and nothing pleases me more than drilling holes and hanging things in my home. My personal style reflects both my biological sex (female) and my gender identity (not too feminine, with a little Annie Hall on the side). I like that I don't fit neatly into any predefined category.

My friend Charles wears his hair cropped close to his head (anything longer than two millimeters and it's time for a haircut), lives in army fatigues and Metallica T-shirts, and has sex with both men and women. His choices reflect his gender role (clean-cut manly), his sexual orientation (he identifies as bisexual), and his fashion sense (military punk).

Sounds good, right? But even if you are a woman who is ready to assert herself in the boardroom, or you're a man who is comfortable staying home and raising kids, or you walk proudly down the street holding your same-sex lover's hand, you might not quite be ready to mess with sex. Men are taught that they are supposed to be the aggressors while women are supposed to wait passively for male sexual attention and then must be talked into having sex. How does that affect same-sex relationships? Sound like some outmoded Victorian morality? Well, it is, but you would be surprised at how these ideas affect even the most liberated of us today.

"It's really hard for me to come, so I always try to tell guys what I like," says Patty, twenty-seven. *"But once I was telling this guy how I liked to be touched, and he got really offended and said I was making him feel really insecure and like he didn't know what to do! He even claimed I was attacking his masculinity!"*

What a tough situation! A woman finally screws up the courage to tell a guy what she needs in bed and gets a negative reaction. I would hazard a guess that it is due to his ideas about how men and women "should" act in bed more than anything inappropriate or hurtful that Patty actually did. And while this is a tricky situation, it is not impossible to overcome. Of course, overcoming will take work on both partners' sides. Maybe this guy needs to be told what to do, but not during sex play. Or maybe Patty could try using different language when giving direction. People are very sensitive when it comes to sex play, and even though it might seem that we are sometimes doing a complicated dance to avoid making someone uncomfortable, or challenging long-held assumptions about gender roles, this is sometimes a dance that needs doing.

Gender Role Models

No matter how liberated our families, gender assumptions are still imposed on us. For example, a family might be very open-minded about duties and roles for boys and girls, making whichever kid is handy set the table or mow the lawn and not delegating these tasks specifically to boys or girls. But they might still insist that a girl not walk home alone at night for safety's sake and not demand this of her younger brother.

Whether this is "just being realistic," as some people would argue, or not, requiring different behaviors for boys and girls contributes to our understanding of ourselves in the world as male or female.

According to Jorge, thirty-seven, the basic messages in his house were different for the girls and the boys: *"My sisters were told: Don't have sex, and if you get pregnant, you will bring shame on the family and we will disown you. I was told: Don't be stupid and get someone pregnant. So it was okay and expected for the boys to have sex, but definitely not the girls."*

Jessica's best childhood friend was her next-door neighbor Jeremy. From the time they were four years old, they had frequent sleepovers, alternating between each other's houses. *"When I was eight years old, I told my father that Jeremy and I were going to have a sleepover that night. My father looked at me sternly and asked, 'Where will you be sleeping?' I knew from his expression that sleeping in Jeremy's room wasn't okay anymore, but I really didn't know why. I felt as though I had done something wrong and that it had to do with Jeremy being a boy and my wanting to sleep in his room, but I really wasn't sure what it was. I ended up sleeping in his sister's room and never had another sleepover in Jeremy's room."* Jessica, now thirty-seven years old, says that *"it was my father's awkwardness, but it became my awkwardness. I couldn't understand what was wrong with what I wanted to do, but I couldn't ask my father. From that time on, there was a barrier between me and my dad about me and guys."*

"I grew up in a house with two stepbrothers who were ten and eleven years older than me, so a lot of my sex education came from listening to them," says Jordan, thirty-two. *"They were all about how great sex was and how they could 'get some pussy' and 'get their rocks off.' Sex was a game, and the goal was to get a girl into bed. They would laugh and 'high-five' if one of them 'scored.' I would laugh along with them—not that I really understood it—and they would say, 'Just wait,*

little brother, someday you'll find out what you're missing.' When I started having sex, I was all about getting some until I realized that what was missing from what my brothers taught me was any idea about giving pleasure, not just getting some."

Yvette, thirty-one, recalls what happened when her sister got pregnant: *"My sister got pregnant when she was seventeen years old, and my father didn't speak to her until after the baby was born. He wouldn't come to the baby shower or celebrate her birthday. He is a very proud man, and he and my mom came here from the Caribbean because they wanted us to have better opportunities. He was so mad and disappointed in her, and he took it personally. It was really hard on her and made him even stricter with the rest of us. There was no way we were bringing any boys home to meet him. After my sister had the baby, one day she heard him bragging about his grandson. She knew that the worst was over, but to this day he doesn't trust any of the guys we date."*

How does growing up in this kind of environment affect our sense of self and our place in the world? The answer is that everyone reacts differently. Some people are very comfortable in the roles that are assigned to them, and some people rebel.

"My father sent me off to college with the following warning: If you have sex, I will break your legs," recalls Jennifer, forty-four, *"and he claimed that he would be able to tell by looking me in the eyes. I came from a Conservative Jewish home. I don't think he would've actually broken my legs, but I wasn't totally sure. I did lose my virginity that first semester to a non-Jewish guy, which was the ultimate sin, and when it was time to go home for Thanksgiving, I was terrified. My friends promised me that there was no way he'd be able to tell, but I was convinced that he would know. All weekend I was waiting for him to notice and say something, but he never did. I wish he had been able to teach me about sex in a positive rather than a threatening way and to accept that I could make good choices for myself. Defying him heightened the thrill of having sex, but it also made it more difficult for me to relax and truly enjoy sex."*

"My cousin Trina was maybe in her late twenties when I was a

*teenager. All anyone in the family could talk about was how she was go-
ing to die a spinster. I was told that women who didn't get married and
have children were a great embarrassment. My parents endlessly asked
me why I didn't have more dates. I was kind of shy and not particularly
popular, and kids at my school didn't really date anyhow. I always felt I
was letting my parents down. I remember lying in bed at night terrified
that I wouldn't get married and that maybe I would be sterile, too. Here
I was, a healthy sixteen-year-old, worrying that my ovaries were dried
up! I honestly doubt the boys in my family ever thought about that!"*
recalls Sabrina, thirty-three.

*"I hated sports. I was pudgy, uncoordinated, and more interested in
math class than sports,"* says Patrick, forty-six. *"This was unacceptable
to my father. He never actually called me a sissy directly, but he definitely
made it clear that he was worried about my teenage masculinity because I
preferred books to balls and couldn't hold a hockey stick to save my life."*

Some of our most potent messages about sexuality and gender roles came from our peers. André's peers were not having
sex but still seemed to have all the answers. André, twenty-eight,
recalls: *"No guy I knew got anywhere near having sex. But despite
this they were all really picky about the kinds of girls they claimed they
would sleep with and what they would do when that moment came. She
had to be built. She had to think he was a god. And he would never go
down on her but was fully expecting blow jobs in return. I sometimes
wonder what these guys' sex lives are like now!"*

On the other hand, Fiona, thirty-nine, got totally different
messages from her peers: *"Girls I knew just did not have sex in high
school. If we suspected a girl was sexually active, we would whisper
about her and would never have been friends with her. I grew up in a really conservative community, and the lines between good girls and bad
girls were clearly drawn."*

Androgyny

The word *androgyny* means "man-woman" and is derived from
the Greek roots *andr* (man) and *gyne* (woman). Androgynous

individuals are those who have integrated aspects of femininity and masculinity into their self-concept and progressed beyond traditional gender roles. Androgynous individuals express whatever behavior seems appropriate in a given situation instead of limiting their response to traditional gender roles. Therefore, androgynous men and women could be assertive or aggressive on the job but tender or nurturing with lovers and/or children.

It has been suggested by sex researchers that androgynous individuals are able to approach life with more flexibility than strongly gender-roled people. Those who are able to transcend traditional gender ideas may be able to function with more comfort and effectiveness in a broader range of situations. Androgynous individuals are able to select from a broad matrix of feminine and masculine behaviors based not on sex role norms, but on what gives them the most personal comfort and satisfaction relative to a given situation. There is also evidence that androgynous men and women have more healthy attitudes toward sexuality than people who are traditionally sex roled.

Truth is, none of us are complete stereotypes of masculine or feminine, and the ways in which we behave with respect to our gender roles will change with time, situation, age, and so on. The following quote from Stephanie Dowrick's book *Intimacy and Solitude* beautifully articulates what gender aspirations should be:

> You may feel locked into society's expectations of someone of your gender. You may experience yourself as someone who is choosing your own way of being. You may be in a relationship with someone of the same gender. You may have swapped the usual gender roles with your opposite-sex partner. Although it may be difficult to transcend your gender, an inner sense of security and flexibility that offers you the opportunity to encourage in yourself the attitudes, feelings and responses that

most appropriately express who you are, without too much regard for whether these conventionally match current gender stereotypes, is attainable. The goal is behaving, thinking, feeling, dreaming, acting, responding in ways which feel true to your own self whether or not this fits conventional expectations of your biological gender.

REFLECTION ON GENDER ROLES

What messages did you get about women and sexuality?

_____

_____

What messages did you get about men and sexuality?

_____

_____

How do you think these messages impacted on your sexuality?

_____

_____

List what ways you fit traditional gender stereotypes and the cultural rules to which you adhere as far as your gender is concerned.

_____

_____

List the ways in which don't you fit traditional gender stereotypes and the cultural rules that you break as far as your gender is concerned.

_____

_____

_____

What are the "shoulds" that drive you sexually (for instance, I should have sex x times per week, I should be able to maintain my erection for at least twenty minutes, I should be able to come every time)?

_____

_____

What roles do you enjoy (for example, being in charge, being subservient) as far as your sexual encounters?

_____

_____

How do you feel about what you have written above?

_____

_____

How might that affect the way you interact sexually with others?

_____

_____

Attraction

Over the years, I have had umpteen crushes and been attracted to classmates, teachers, co-workers, men, women, celebrities—the list is varied and long. When I was eleven years old, I was a card-carrying member of the David Cassidy Fan Club. David awakened my nascent prepubescent sexual longing and desire; I had 750 pictures of him on my walls (yes, I counted) and would lull myself to sleep each night fantasizing about how one day I would meet him and he would fall in love with me. My fantasies were elaborate and creative. So powerful was this attraction that I would tape-record *The Partridge Family* each Friday night and play the tape all week long just to hear his voice (this was in the days before TiVo). Even now my heart skips a beat when I hear the song "I Think I Love You."

What was it about David that gave me butterflies in my stomach? His adorable shag haircut? His slightly crooked teeth? His puka-shell necklace?

What was it about a particular person that set your heart a-flutter? Why did you get tongue-tied in front of the girl your friends described as "gawky with glasses who smells like pickles"? Why do gorgeous supermodels date scrawny rock stars? Who can explain attraction? Sometimes obvious things attract you to a person, like hair color, height, butt, breasts, quirky laugh, dark skin, or John Travolta chin. As one famous sex researcher, Helen Singer Kaplan, says, "It all starts with desire."

But desire can be tricky. We get messages about whom we "should" be attracted to that may be in conflict with the attraction(s) we "actually" feel—such as that toward someone of the same sex or another ethnic or religious group. For instance, thirteen-year-old boys are not *supposed* to be attracted to Mr. Williams, the cute young math teacher, but everyone nods conspiratorially when the thirteen-year-old girls confess their crushes on the same Mr. Williams. Though we sure have come a long way since 1967 when interracial marriage was finally legalized in America, a lot of people are still uncomfortable with dating between people whose skin tones are different. All of these issues can play a role in choosing partners, as demonstrated by the experiences described below:

"I lost my virginity to a guy when I was fourteen. I felt attracted to men but never doubted that someday I would be with a woman. My best friend and I had already talked about sleeping with each other when we were ready. She and I would curl up on the bed together and sleep all cuddled up. Sometimes we would kiss and as we got older would start making out. So I always just imagined that one day I'd

sleep with her and get it out of my system. But we both continued dating men and sleeping with them and never ended up doing more than kissing.

"Then at eighteen my friend took me to my first gay club, and before we left his dorm room I said, 'I'm going to hook up with a girl tonight.' We went and were dancing for a while when a really cute girl approached me. I totally backed away, and she got the hint. Then a few minutes later I looked across the room and saw a girl so sexy that I knew she was the girl I had to hook up with. So we did end up hooking up that night, and shortly after she became my first girlfriend for ten months.

"She had already been with women, and when we were having sex she would basically just fool around with me. But I realized the time was approaching when I would have to at least give it a shot. So about two months into our relationship, I ventured 'down there' and was so completely shocked. I was pretty sexually comfortable with men by that point in my life, but I really had no idea how to be with a woman. It may sound stupid, but I expected her body to be like mine . . . and that's when I discovered women have different vaginas! I ended up being just fine and developed a fabulous sexual relationship with my girlfriend.

"After my first experiences with a woman, I was no less attracted to men, but I found out how strong my attraction to women really was. Now I identify as bisexual and really feel equally inclined to sleep with women as I do men. Everyone's always saying, 'Come on, you have to like one more than the other. . . . Which do you prefer to sleep with, men or women?' And I have to go through the same speech over and over again, trying to explain to people that I truly love men and women the same." Amy, twenty-four.

"I really shared my vagina with a girl at college. She was gentle and caring, and we fell in 'love' for a time. We masturbated in front of each other, and this turned us on. We never made love, but the feelings we had for this were very strong." Steph, fifty-one.

Sexual Orientation

*W*hat is straight and what is gay? Basically, a straight person is someone who is sexually attracted to people of the opposite sex—people who have genitals that are different from their own. A gay or lesbian person is turned on by those whose sex organs are the same as theirs, and bisexuals are sexually drawn to both.

Clearly it's more complicated than that. Sexual orientation is not the same as sexual behavior. A man who has sex with men may or may not consider himself to be gay. A women who identifies as a lesbian may have sex with both men and women. Someone who considers herself straight may have experimented sexually with women. At one time or another, most of us have had some attraction to those who have genitals like ours. It is not helpful or accurate for you to label someone as straight, gay, lesbian, or bisexual because of whom he or she has sex with. Sexual orientation is a *self-identity,* and whether or not someone chooses to label him- or herself (or, if the person identifies as transgender, "hirself") is really not important (except if the person isn't being honest with you).

You can be attracted to anyone you like, but you have a choice about how you identify. You can decide to act or not act on your attraction, and there may be both negatives and positives in that decision. For example, you may choose not to act on your same-sex attractions in order to maintain your religious ties, acceptance in your community, and/or family approval. That may be fine, but there may be costs associated with that choice, such as the loss of a partner to whom you are attracted, feeling untrue to yourself, or an inability to be authentic. But that's for you to decide.

Think about attractions you have had or currently have to boyfriends, girlfriends, lovers, crushes, husbands, wives, and so

on. What about them is/was attractive to you? List those qualities below. You may want to list specific people and specific
qualities for each person or just generate a list of qualities
(such as red hair, funky shoes, married and unavailable, tattoo,
intelligence, neck wattle, great laugh, and so on).

_____

_____

_____

What do you notice about your attractions to others?

_____

_____

_____

In what ways have your attractions changed over the years?

_____

_____

_____

What aspects of your attractions have remained constant?
What about these aspects have been appealing over time?

_____

_____

_____

How do you identify as far as your sexual orientation? Has that
changed over time? Do you see that changing in the future?

_____

_____

How we present ourselves, to whom we are attracted, and with
whom we choose to have sex are products of our biological sex,

GENDER ROLE, SEX, GENDER IDENTITY AND SEXUAL ORIENTATION MATRIX								
Biological Sex	Female			Intersex		Male		
Gender Identity	Female			Transgender		Male		
Gender Role	Feminine (Barbie)	←――――――――――――――――――→					Masculine (Rambo)	
Sexual Orientation	Lesbian	Gay	Straight	Questioning	Bisexual	Queer	Pansexual	Asexual

our gender identity, and our sexual orientation. Choosing from each row of the chart shown here can help to form a more accurate, comprehensive description of your sexuality. For example, someone may have a penis and testicles, identify as transgender, display socially constructed feminine characteristics, and choose to be sexually intimate with both men and women. How an individual chooses to put together these identities may change based on age, time of life, season of the year, experiences, and other life circumstances. Some people struggle with their multiple identities. For example, someone who is female and identifies as a woman may feel conflicted about her attraction to both men and women. She may choose to identify as bisexual but act only upon her attractions to men. A man who identifies as a man and subscribes to a masculine gender role may have sex with men but not identify as gay. You cannot judge from someone's behavior the entire range of his or her sexuality. Even creating a matrix like the one shown in the chart can be limiting in describing sexuality.

Chapter 5

LOVING THE SKIN THAT YOU'RE IN

Appreciating Your Body and Its Sexual Capacity

* * *

Self-acceptance is hard for many of us. There is a voice inside
that is constantly judging, first ourselves and then others. . . .
Because we have learned to believe negativity is more realistic, it
appears more real than any positive voice. Once we begin to
replace negative thinking with being realistic, negative thinking is
absolutely disenabling. When we are positive we not only accept
and affirm ourselves, we are able to affirm and accept others.
—From the bell hooks treatise *all about love*

I hate my boobs. My penis is too small. Why did I have to
be cursed with cellulite?! Why can't I have six-pack abs?!
Sound familiar? Even if you haven't uttered these complaints,
it is very likely you dislike something about your body.

According to Aline P. Zoldbrod, in her 1998 book *Sex Smart:*
How Your Childhood Shaped Your Sexual Life and What You Can Do

About It, since the mind is your primary sex organ, "your nega-tive feelings about your body constrain your bodily enjoyment. Factors like the amount and distribution of the body hair you have, your height, your weight, or the size and shape of your breast or penis do not determine how sexually responsive you are. But any negative feelings you have about your bodily char-acteristics put a damper on your ability to be uninhibited."

To be sexually healthy, you must develop an appreciation of how your body looks and feels, knowledge about how it works, appropriate boundaries around who, what, when, where, and in what way you are sexually approached, and the encouragement to explore your sexuality.

No matter what your body looks like, the more comfortable you are with it, the better sex play will be with another person. Why is that? Simply, when we like and trust ourselves, it is a lot easier to be open, free, and experimental. If you are constantly trying to maneuver yourself so your cellulite is hidden, or if you let a partner see you only when you are erect because you think your penis looks too small when it is flaccid, then you are misus-ing precious energy that could be spent on pleasuring.

Many of us are dissatisfied with our appearance. It can be tough to be satisfied when every reality TV show and popular magazine is encouraging us to lose fifty pounds and undergo plastic surgery to cure any and all unhappiness.

Face it: Most of us don't fit the current standard of beauty or brawn, whether it's our size, shape, skin color, hair color, or whatever. The average person is neither supersvelte nor built like a brick house, does not have voluptuous Angelina Jolie or Mick Jagger lips, and is most likely not sporting bodacious breasts or a bulging manhood. So should all average-looking people throw in the towel and say sex isn't for them until they go on *Extreme Makeover*? Obviously not. Media and other cul-tural messages are not the only factors that influence body image. The appropriateness and amount of touch we experienced as children, our physical abilities, and assessments of our body (usually unsolicited) by family members, peers, and other community members all played a significant role in how we, as adults, feel about our bodies.

Lucas, twenty-six, grew up in Germany and thinks that *"because of this I have a different body consciousness than a lot of Americans. People are a lot more open about their bodies, and I think overall this makes us more comfortable and happier about how we look."*

Carmen, forty-six, recalls how her mother's self-perceived disfigurement from cancer had such a key effect on her own sense of body: *"My mom had a mastectomy when I was seven years old, and from that time on, I never saw her body. I knew she was ashamed of it. As I got older, I got more curious about what it looked like and asked her if I could see. She told me that it would upset me and she didn't want me to see it. I always pictured it as horribly scarred and ugly. When I was about fifteen years old and we were away on a trip, she came out of the bathroom without her bra on. She saw me, covered her chest, and ran into the bathroom. I saw it. It was really nothing—no scarring, no horror—just flat skin. I couldn't get over how 'nothing' it was. Yet to her it was so traumatic and disfiguring, the worst thing that could have happened. We never spoke about what happened, but I realized that it wasn't how she looked that was so horrifying to her, it was the loss of her breast and what that meant."*

"My dad was always telling my mom how fat she was," says Erik, thirty-two. *"It would make me really angry. He watched everything she ate and would give her a hard time about eating anything fattening. He would take food out of her hand and say, 'You don't need that, you're fat enough.' I would stick up for her and say, 'She's fine just the way she is.' He eventually left us, and Mom was heartbroken. I swore that I would never be that way with my wife. It makes me sick to admit this, but when I see girls who are fat, there's this voice in the back of my head that judges them, just like my dad judged my mom. I hate that I*

think this way because I saw how it destroyed her self-esteem and I wouldn't wish that on anyone."

Maria, twenty-six, grew up with her mother and grand-mother, both of whom immigrated to the United States from Mexico: *"To my mother and grandmother, being heavier meant being healthy. Thin was sickly. But that was not how it was in my school. What was acceptable for my body size and shape in my family was what I got teased about in school. It was so confusing, and when the boys called me 'lardass' and I went home crying, my grandmother would hold me in her arms and rock me and tell me how beautiful I was."*

Pubies and Boobies and Pimples, Oh My!

*P*uberty, the time period during which all those wonderfully awkward emotional, hormonal, and physical changes that en-compass your sexual development occur, is a milestone on the sexual journey of your life. All of a sudden you're sporting breasts or popping boners. Your voice breaks unceremoniously as you self-consciously talk to that cute girl who has a smatter-ing of pimples on her forehead. Whether you were an early or late bloomer, whether it was hell on earth filled with disconcert-ing changes or a blissful time filled with exciting changes, you were undoubtedly affected by puberty. Many people still have lingering issues or feelings of physical inadequacy that come from this time in their life, often left over from insensitive (and sometimes cruel) peer or familial ridicule:

"My brothers teased me about getting breasts, so I knew that they were scrutinizing my body as it developed. I took to wearing oversize clothes and avoiding being around them in a bathing suit. One day my oldest brother made a comment about 'wasn't it time that I lost my baby fat.' I was mortified. It was the comment that put me over the edge and was the start of many years of eating disorders. I'm much better now, but my eating and my body are a constant struggle. About three years ago I

confronted my brother about what he said—he has a daughter now who's almost eleven years old and I'd hate to see her have to go through what I went through—but he laughed it off. He said he was just teasing me and it's not his fault I got so messed up." Clara, thirty-nine.

"I grew boobs before anyone else, and I really think it made people think that I was doing things I wasn't. Boys would accidentally bump into me, and the girls would say things about me behind my back. I started wearing really big shirts, but it didn't really help much." Melissa, twenty-nine.

"When I was thirteen my friend Jay was practically a man! I mean, he was thirteen, too, but he was big and had chest hair and seemed so much older. It was kind of intimidating because my voice hadn't even started changing yet." Tyrone, thirty-three.

Mario, now twenty-two, says that his biggest fear was getting naked with a girl: *"I didn't have pubic hair until I was about seventeen or so, and my penis looked the same as it had when I was a kid. I was tall enough, but for some reason that part of puberty just wasn't kicking in. I was terrified that if I ever got together with a girl, she would laugh at me and tell everyone that I was actually a baby trapped in a teenager's body."*

"All I wanted was to grow! I was one of the shortest kids in school and was terrified that I would stay that way forever. It doesn't matter how many times adults can tell you you're a late bloomer, when you are desperately waiting for something like that time seems to stand still." Thomas, forty-five.

"Did you ever read the book Are You There, God? It's Me, Margaret? *Well, I was like Margaret, begging God for boobs and my period. Only thing is, Margaret gets hers at like twelve or thirteen, while I had to wait until I was sixteen! Once I got it I would get these terrible cramps every month and have to miss a day of school. I felt disgusting!"* Patrice, thirty-six.

Time Marches On

*U*nless you are a statue on display in the House of Wax, you will find that your body is constantly changing. Monthly hormonal surges impact your physical and mental state of being, your weight fluctuates on a daily basis, gravity affects your height (you're taller in the morning than you are in the evening), and despite a proliferation of antiaging products and surgical procedures currently touted in the media, you just can't stop the march of time. While aging is accompanied by some very real sexual changes that require adjustments in sexual expectations, it can also be liberating. As my eighty-five-year-old Aunt Rose once told me, "My sixties were the best years because I finally didn't give a rat's ass about what anyone else thought about my looks."

Nina, fifty-four, says, *"I am more self-conscious now that I am older. Having not been with a partner or a husband in a long time, I have to mentally remind myself that I am beautiful. I have not taken off my clothes in front of a man in two years, and I need to reaffirm how I feel about myself before I do that. Although now I know how to play up my sexiness differently than I did when I was younger. If you know how to do that, then you can still be sexy at any age without looking ridiculous."*

Jerry, thirty-four, says, *"I never really thought about what I looked like until I started balding at twenty-five. Then I became really self-conscious and with that less confident."*

Francie, twenty-seven, talks about her self-image after having a baby: *"Shortly after we had our son, my husband and I split up, and it did a real number on my ego. But a year or so later, I met a new guy and he made me feel really sexy, even though my body looked a little different than it had a few years before. He really liked the fact that I was a mom, and that made me feel comfortable and sexy."*

Eric W. Johnson, in his book *Older and Wiser: Wit, Wisdom, and Spirited Advice from the Older Generation,* collected the thoughts of older adults about aging and sexuality. Here is what some had to say:

"*Old age is honorable, beautiful, natural, and still full of possibilities.*" Sixty-eight-year-old woman.

"*I'm waiting with bated breath—when will I feel old?*" Eighty-six-year-old man.

"*My wife and I have been married thirty-four years, and I have the feeling that we achieved more happy physical adjustment during the past three or four years than ever before, a sort of new awakening to quiet, deep joy.*" Seventy-four-year-old man.

"*I think it's disgusting that these old people go around looking for sex. When you get flabby and dry, you ought to stop trying to be young and accept your age and quit looking for sex. Memories are enough.*" Sixty-nine-year-old woman.

"*Sex over sixty-five? No objection, except that too much is made of the subject. . . . Physical closeness, tenderness, and affection (expressed in many ways) are so much more rewarding and meaningful than intercourse.*" Seventy-four-year-old woman.

The Skin You're In

*M*arylin, twenty-four, says, "*People tell me I'm hot, and I guess technically I can see it, but I would never get naked with a guy because I am worried that he'll see things on me that will turn him off, like if I haven't shaved that day or if I'm feeling fat. No one's ever said anything mean to me, but the thought of what they might think makes me really scared.*"

On the other hand, Adam, twenty-six, who is a self-described "shlub," feels great in bed: "*I don't look like a movie star by any means and have been balding for years, which I know isn't considered the sexiest thing for a young guy, but I don't really care. If I'm with someone, I figure they want to be there and aren't expecting Brad Pitt when I take my shirt off. I love being naked, I love trying new positions,* and I really just assume that unless I hear different my partner is as turned on as I am."

Not everyone wants a partner who is a perfect physical specimen. Ollie, thirty-one, says, "I'm just not into big boobs. My girlfriend is less than an A cup, and that is great. I just wouldn't know what to do with any more boob!"

Lauren, twenty-seven, thinks that "a guy who is too pretty is boring. And I know it is a stereotype, but I think it makes him look like he would be lazy in bed. All I see is lazy, and I just fall asleep. I get really excited by a guy who seems rough around the edges."

"I might think someone is attractive, but if we can't have a good conversation, then I am not normally interested," says Francis, thirty-three. "The first time I saw Margot, I didn't think she was very attractive. But we hung out for a few hours and talked, and by the end of the night we had made a date for the next day. Over time I realized I was finding her better and better looking, and now I have to remind myself I thought she was kind of plain when we first met."

"I love girls with big butts." Reggie, twenty-seven.

Writer Rachel Kramer Bussel relates,

> Nothing gets me hotter than a nice, big belly, perhaps not so surprising since I consider James Gandolfini and Monica Lewinsky both people I'd fuck in a heartbeat. Actually, it doesn't have to be all that big, but the belly (and never "stomach," because that word just kills my libido right there) is so soft and curvy, reminiscent of the ass or a breast but softer and more sensitive, like the inner thigh. The belly is a totally underappreciated erogenous zone and is also perfectly poised between the nipples and genitals, so you can linger there, licking and teasing, making someone wonder what exactly you're going to do next. Bellies are sexy to me because they are so soft and sensual, tender and juicy, they make me want to

touch and taste them, and if there were a contest for giving belly blow jobs, I'm sure I would win. Washboard stomachs make me want to run screaming; flat stomachs are like flat chests to me, they just do nothing for me. But curvy, pillowy bellies that I can lay my head on, that I can rub up against, tease and tickle and bite and lick, tweak gently when I'm busy doing something else, get me every time. They don't have to be huge, I'm not a size queen about this, but they have to somehow be there, and the person has to like, or at least tolerate, me fawning over theirs.

"I think I am attracted to different things in guys and girls," Simone says, twenty-eight. *"But one thing I am attracted to in both is confidence. Confidence really goes a long way!"*

Most people don't expect their partners to look like porn or movie stars. Granted, few people like a poorly groomed, hygienically challenged slob, but taking care of your body and avoiding sex because you think that no one could be turned on once they see your stretch marks are two totally different things.

Unless you have some specific reason to believe your partner is lying when he or she tells you that you're beautiful and sexy, why question it? Wouldn't you rather have sex with someone imperfect in appearance (by society's standards) but avidly into you and enthusiastic than someone who looks more like a pinup but is so hung up about body image that he or she can't relax or focus on pleasing you?

Erica, thirty-nine, recalls, *"One day, when I was feeling particularly unattractive—adult acne breakout, short haircut that I hated—my boyfriend came home with a new camera. Our relationship was not great at the time, and we hadn't been having sex much at all. Anyway, he started taking pictures of me and wanted me to take off my shirt. I took off my clothes and got into it, too, posing. It was so erotic. He really got into it, telling me how hot I was, taking close-ups of my vagina and breasts. It helped me feel great about my body."*

REFLECTION: BODY IMAGE

Describe your most vivid memories of puberty.

_____

_____

_____

Describe a time when you were teased about some aspect of your appearance.

_____

_____

_____

_____

How have these experiences affected the way you view your body?

_____

_____

_____

_____

ACTIVITY: MY BODY MAP*

Draw a picture of both the front and the back of your body in the space below. Be sure to include your features (eyes, genitals, scars,

---

*Adapted from the "Draw Your Body Map" exercise in Aline P. Zoldbrod's wonderful book *Sex Smart* (New Harbinger Publications, 1998).

moles, piercings, and so on). Using a pen, circle the parts of your body that you like and put an X through the parts that you dislike.

What do you notice about where you placed the circles and where you placed an X?

_____

_____

What are your favorite body parts?

_____

What are your least favorite body parts?

_____

What prevents you from appreciating this part of your body?

_____

_____

Now, using red, yellow, and green pens or markers, make a dot on the body parts that fit the categories below.
- Red = I never like to be touched here.
- Yellow = I may or may not want you to touch me here, depending on the situation and how I feel.
- Green = I always like to be touched here.

What color predominates? In which area? Why do you think that is?

_____

_____

_____

Under what conditions would it be okay for someone to touch the yellow areas?

_____

_____

Describe the connection between the parts of your body that have circles and X's and those that have red, yellow, or green dots.

_____

_____

What do some people say about their own bodies after doing the exercise above?

"I don't want anyone touching my feet or sucking on my toes. I don't think my feet are attractive, and I don't think it feels good." Annette, fifty-four.

"I'm okay with someone seeing me naked from the front," says Sienna, thirty-nine, *"but I'm really self-conscious about having someone see my butt in the light of day. I'll only back out of a room or wrap a towel or blanket around me if I'm exiting."*

Theodore, forty-two, says, *"I have an extra nipple on my chest. I hate it. I feel freaky."*

The truth is, everyone dislikes something about their general physical appearance or has some body part that they wish could be bigger or smaller or softer or smoother or shorter or longer, but if you're going to grow, and be more comfortable sexually, you will need to figure out a way to make peace with the parts of your body that, however imperfect, make it unique.

ACTIVITY: A JOURNEY THROUGH TIME: MY BODY AND ME*

Just as researching and recording a family history can help you understand and take pride in your heritage, writing your unique body history can help you feel more accepting and appreciative of your body.

Directions:

- On a piece of paper turned horizontally, draw a line across the center of the page, leaving about a half-inch margin on either side. You may need to add other pages, so you'll want to allow room to attach them to one another. Leave plenty of space to write along the line.
- On the left-hand side of the line, write your birthday.
- Think about your physical development and how your body has changed over your lifetime.
- Record as many changes as you can remember through the years. Try to place these changes in some sort of chronological order.
- Include physical changes that enabled you to master new skills and abilities or disabilities that became milestones in your life (such as being able to swim across the pool, getting your first pair of eyeglasses, your first gray pubic hair).

---

*This activity is adapted from "Your Body's Historical Timeline" in the book *Sex Matters for Women* by Sallie Foley, Sally A. Kope, and Dennis P. Sugrue (Guilford Press, 2002).

- Include sexual changes in your body, such as when you started your period or when you started menopause, and your first orgasm (if you've had one).
- Some changes are simply the discovery of a quality that had always been present. If you are a person of color, for example, you may remember the first time in which the color of your skin became the focus of an exchange. If you were taller than your peers, perhaps you never paid attention to that until someone commented on it.
- Record temporary or permanent changes in your body that were a result of either personal choice or circumstance, such as pregnancy, getting a tattoo, or weight fluctuations.
- Keep noting changes up until your present age. The timeline may take several days to complete. You may notice clusters of changes around developmental milestones such as puberty.

For each change that you recorded, ask yourself the following questions:

- Did I receive information or did anyone talk to me about this change?
- How did I react to this body change?
- In what way did this change impact on my sexuality?

After you have completed the timeline, answer the questions below:

What stands out for you in this timeline?

_____

_____

_____

What were the positive aspects of your body's growing and changing?

_____

_____

What surprised you about this timeline?

_____

_____

Other reflections and comments:

_____

_____

IMPROVING YOUR BODY IMAGE

You need a small flashlight preferably the size of a pen and a dark room. Quickly point the light at some portion of your partner's body. With the focus of the light, examine that part of his or her body. Turn off the light and take a moment to feel that body part in the dark. What are the differences you notice about it when you lose your sight as a sense? What do you notice when you are able to "see" it? Repeat this exercise until you have examined all parts of your partner's body, inch by inch. The advantage to this exercise is that throughout it, you still have the privacy of being in the dark yet the benefits of light. After spending several hours exploring each other's bodies this way, you could vary the assignment by using the flashlight to play doctor. In this version, the flashlight is used for the examination of your partner's body parts. This is important because the doctor needs some way to make sure nothing is "seriously wrong." Finish the doctor's examination with your hands, mouth, and sex toys.

—Developed by Alex Robboy, LSW

Chapter 6

VOYAGE TO THE LAND OF VULVAS AND VAGINAS

What You Need to Know About Female Genitals

✳ ✳ ✳

In Tantric Hinduism, the word for vagina also means sacred place. It is emblematic of all creative action, and its receptivity is not regarded as passive, but as energizing, empowering.
—Alexandra Jacoby, artist, creator of
www.vaginaverite.com

The next part of our journey takes us on a voyage to the land of vulvas and vaginas. When it comes to their vaginas, many women still shy away form talk about "down there."

In a survey sponsored by the Association of Reproductive Health Professionals and conducted by the Harris Poll, a random sample of women ages eighteen to forty-four were canvassed about their attitudes on women's health. Among the responses: seventy-three percent said that the vagina is a shocking topic, less than half have ever performed a self-exam of their vagina, one in four had not looked at her vagina in the past year, and only one in ten said that there is no shame in having discussions about vaginas.

Interestingly, women say that their significant others' perception of their vagina is that it is sexy, beautiful, or amazing. But they themselves may not be in agreement with that assessment, as evidenced by the following quotes from women:

"I looked at my vagina once, and the inside is totally a different color from the outside! I don't think it is supposed to look like that, and I wonder if people look at me and think I have a disease." Angelique, twenty-two.

"I'm concerned that I'm not tight enough anymore. I've had two babies, and even though my partner hasn't said anything, I am really worried that it feels different for him and he isn't enjoying sex as much as he did before we had kids." Val, thirty-seven.

"I don't ever want anyone to go down on me because I am worried

What Do You Call It?

China	kooter	*piciachi*	big montana	*punani*
fotze	flower power	box	pishy	pus pus
fickloch	gwaff	tender trap	sinkhole	honeypot
möse	hole	origin of the	ax wound	you
sugar dish	flower	world	va-jay-jay	hootch
cock socket	twat	schmoony	cookie	snatch
cave	food	*cosita*	vagina	fur burger
soft spot	love hole	*panocha*	pussy	bearded clam
sweet spot	*la petite fleur*	two big lips	cunt	
danger zone	yin-yang	little bird	beaver	
garage	coochie	*shushka*	love-tunnel	—From Rutgers
private doorway	kitty	grand opening	woo woo	University human
twa	padaka	man in the boat	va-jj	sexuality class

that I smell bad. The few times it has happened I've really liked it, but no matter what I do, I just smell kind of strong." Veronica, thirty.

"I'm really hairy, but every time I try to shave I get a terrible rash and ingrown hairs. I've tired creams and waxing, but nothing really works. My boyfriend loves the clean-shaven look, but there is no way I will ever have a cute, smooth vagina. Sometimes I just look down and think I look really ugly, all rashy and hairy." Andrea, nineteen.

One of my favorite vagina Web sites, www.vaginaverite.com, was started by Alexandra Jacoby in response to the following conversation:

"It started one day when a friend of mine asked me apropos of nothing: Did I like the way my vagina looked? As I answered, I realized that I had never really taken a good look at it and that other than a bit of porn, I hadn't really seen any other women's vaginas. I was pretty sure that they were all different but had nothing to point to when talking with my friend, who clearly thought there was something wrong with how hers looked. What could I say?"

Landscape

*T*he first and most important concept in V-land is that the vulva and the vagina are not one and the same. The *vagina* is an internal organ that connects a woman's outer sex organs with the *cervix* and *uterus* via a stretchable passage that is typically four to five inches long. The vagina has soft, moist walls and is lined by a smooth surface that contains many mucous glands. The *vulva* is the term for all the parts of a woman's body that make up her external sex organs. This includes the *clitoris,* the *clitoral hood,* the *labia,* the opening to the vagina, and the *Bartholin's glands,* which produce some lubrication during sex play.

A lot of women worry that their vulvas are not normal, which may be because they have never seen their own vulva, much less another vulva. Maybe the only vulva you've seen is the hairless, pink, and perfectly symmetrical vulva found in most adult magazines and pornography. Most women's vulvas just don't look like this. No two vulvas are exactly alike, just as no two faces are exactly alike. Every woman's vulva is unique, with a distinctive look, taste, and smell.

Vulvas can range in color from light pink to bluish black. The outer and inner labia (lips) are often a different color. Labia come in all shapes, sizes, and colors. You may have been taught the terms *labia majora* and *labia minora* to describe the inner and outer lips. These terms are actually inaccurate and can lead to some concern for women because they imply that the outer lips should be bigger than the inner lips. While the outer lips tend to be made up of fattier tissue and covered in hair, the inner lips are often longer and protrude from between their hosts. It is perfectly normal to have one lip that is bigger or longer than the other.

The crowning glory of the vulva is pubic hair (or, as my godson calls it, "vagina fuzz"), which can be curly or straight, dense or sparse. Some women shave it, wax it, use depilatory cream, or dye it (Why, yes, I am a natural blonde!). Pubic hair can extend up to the belly button, over the labia, back up around the *anus,* and down the thighs. Or it can simply provide a small patch over the *mons pubis,* the mound of flesh directly over the labia.

Pubic hair serves many functions, including capturing a woman's odor, which increases the scent of *pheromones,* the sex signals that we unknowingly send out to attract partners. Another function is aesthetics. There is absolutely no hygienic reason women should feel the need to groom, remove, or even trim their pubic hair. Some people find pubic hair a big turn-on and view it as an indication of sexual maturity. Others, however, find minimal hair to be a turn-on.

VULVAR SELF-EXAM

Looking at your vulva is not just a good way to get to know yourself better, it can be a vital tool in taking care of your health. Like any other part of your body, the vulva can get infected, and early treatment tends to be most successful. If you discover something, consult your medical provider.

Examining your vulva involves a handheld mirror, some physical flexibility, and finding a comfortable, well-lit place during a time you know you won't be disturbed. Hold the mirror in one hand. Use the other hand to separate your labia so you can get a good view of all parts of the vulva. You are looking for new moles, warts, or growths as well as areas of pigmentation that may look white, red, or dark and spots where there is pain, inflammation, or itching. Check for bumps under the surface of the skin by lightly pressing your fingers over the entire vulva.

How will you know if this mole is new or has always been there? If you do a self-exam once a month, you will know your vulva like the back of your hand.

Size Matters

There is a lot of misinformation about vagina size and shape. Some people think that a vagina needs to be very small and "tight" to be pleasurable for someone's partner. Others fear that vagina penetration will be painful because their vagina is not large enough to accommodate a partner or other object. But the truth of the matter is, there is not one size that all vaginas should be. The vagina is a stretchable canal lined with muscular folds called *ruggae*. It serves as the birth canal and the passage for menstrual fluid. It is also the organ of vaginal intercourse, where a penis or dildo can be inserted during vaginal sex. The vaginal canal extends back about four to six inches and ends in the bottom of the uterus, otherwise known as the cervix. When a woman is sexually aroused, her vagina actually lengthens! This happens as the uterus tips back and the *ruggae* stretch out. Contrary to popular belief, the vagina is not a never-ending void. Unless something is inserted into the vagina, it actually lies closed. So the vagina should be thought of as a *potential* space rather than a permanent opening.

Care and Feeding of Vulvas and Vaginas

Healthy women experience regular vaginal discharge, which is called *leukorrhea*. Typical vaginal discharge tends to have a distinctive, but not unpleasant, odor that can vary from sweet to musky—it's a woman's personal fragrance. Vaginal scent can be affected by many things, including

- Pregnancy—high estrogen levels result in more abundant vaginal secretions.
- Sweat—active women and women who perspire more easily may have problems with chronic dampness.
- Stress—life's tensions can make you sweat excessively in the vaginal area.
- Medication—antibiotics can affect the pH of the vagina.
- Hormonal fluctuation—most women have a sweeter smell in the first half of their menstrual cycle, when estrogen predominates, and a muskier smell after ovulation, when progesterone takes over.
- Infection—yeast infections, vaginitis, and bacterial vaginosis can affect vaginal pH.
- Diet—what you eat may affect the taste and smell of your vaginal secretions (such as spicy food or changing from a meat-eating to a vegetarian diet).

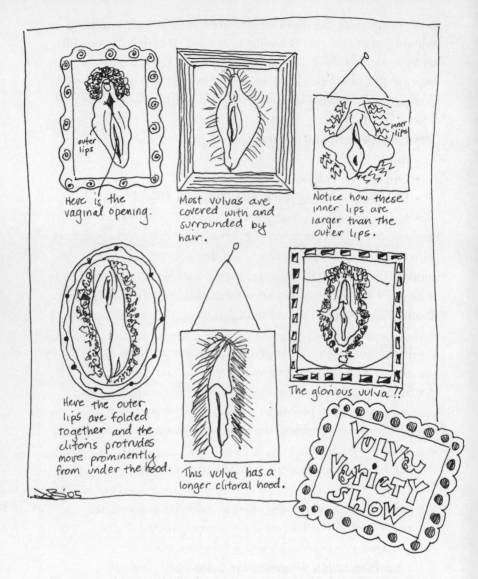

Here is the vaginal opening.

Most vulvas are covered with and surrounded by hair.

Notice how these inner lips are larger than the outer lips.

Here the outer lips are folded together and the clitoris protrudes more prominently from under the hood.

This vulva has a longer clitoral hood.

The glorious vulva!!

Vulva Variety Show

Normal vaginal discharges are either thick and whitish or slippery and clear and change according to the menstrual cycle. For example, when a woman is ovulating her discharge may seem tackier (stickier) than at other times of the month. However, if a woman notices that her discharge is foamy, that the odor changes or becomes unpleasant, or that she has itching or burning, then she may have *vaginitis,* an irritation in the vagina.

Vaginitis can be caused by a number of things, including an overgrowth of bacteria, sexually transmitted infections, allergies, and irritants. Following are common symptoms of vaginitis:

- Changes in color, quantity, or texture of the vaginal fluid.
- Unpleasant odors.
- Bleeding, spotting, or bloody discoloration.
- Itching and/or burning of the vagina or vulva.

A healthy vagina does not need to be specially cleaned. In fact, much like an oven, the vagina is self-cleaning. Products such as douches, hygiene sprays, deodorant tampons, and so on can actually harm the natural pH of the vagina and lead to inflammation and discomfort. Douching by inserting a liquid solution into the vagina in an effort to eradicate unpleasant odor can actually strip the vagina of healthy bacteria and cause infections!

While douching is not a good idea, washing the vulva daily with soap and water is a welcome practice. The vulva is made up of various skin folds that can trap vaginal discharge (or *vegma,* my word for the female version of *smegma*), urine, and, if you are wiping the wrong way, even feces. These may not be something your lover wants to encounter during oral sex. So wash among the folds of the lips, under the clitoral hood, and around the anus.

Pleasurable Moments for Vulvas and Vaginas

C-Spots and G-Spots

When it comes to erogenous zones, any body part (including the nipples, earlobes, and elbows) can be sexually sensitive. But while people have different preferences for how and where they

THE DON'TS OF DOUCHING

A recent report indicates that douching may delay conception in women trying to get pregnant. It's unclear exactly how this happens, but researchers
have found that women who douched were up to 50 percent less likely to
become pregnant each month they tried to conceive. Overall, women who
douched were 30 percent less likely to become pregnant each month they
tried to conceive. *This does not make douching a good form of contracep-
tion.* Research has shown that douching pushes bacteria up the reproductive
tract, which can cause dangerous pelvic inflammatory disease, an inflammation of the pelvic area that can lead to permanent infertility.

are touched, for most women the clitoris is, without question, a
main site of sexual pleasure.

The clitoris is located in the vulva between the inner labia
lips. These lips attach over the clitoris to form the *prepuce,* a pro-
tective hood or foreskin. The clitoris looks a little bit like the tip
of your nose, and like the vulva itself, the clitoris is subject to a
great deal of variety. Some women's clitorises protrude from
between their lips, others remain hidden until arousal; but rest
assured, all women are born with this pleasure center.

The clitoris (or c-spot) is extremely sensitive to touch and is
equivalent in many ways to the head of a penis, with roughly
the same amount of nerve endings. This is not surprising, since
they both start out from the same tissue. Not only do they share
a sensitive head, but both organs also have a shaft that fills with
blood and becomes erect with sexual excitement. This sensitivity can mean that some women really enjoy direct clitoral stimulation while others need a more indirect touch.

Unlike the penis, however, most of the clitoris is not visible because the shaft of the clitoris extends back into the body, where it wraps around to surround the opening of the vagina. So the lower two-thirds of the vagina are the most sensitive (something to keep in mind when inserting a finger or other object). I like to call the clitoris "little grasshopper," because, as the picture below shows, it looks like one.

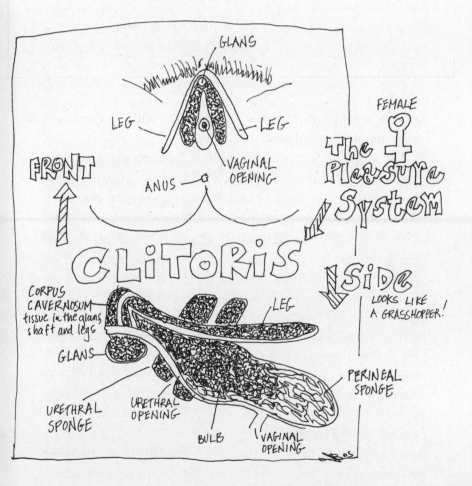

GLANS

LEG — — LEG

FRONT

ANUS — VAGINAL OPENING

FEMALE

The Pleasure System

CLITORIS

SIDE
LOOKS LIKE A GRASSHOPPER!

CORPUS CAVERNOSUM tissue in the glans, shaft and legs

LEG

GLANS

PERINEAL SPONGE

URETHRAL SPONGE

URETHRAL OPENING

BULB

VAGINAL OPENING

Many women have clitoral stories about improper handling of their c-spot:

"When I was seventeen years old I had a hot and passionate romance with my boyfriend, but I just couldn't bring myself to tell him that when he rubbed my clit it felt like he was trying to remove an ink spot. I worried that there would be nothing left after we were done fooling around or that he would do permanent damage. I never got up the courage to tell him, even though it hurt, and I wondered for many years if the extreme sensitivity in my clitoris was due to some damage done by him." LaToya, twenty-eight.

"I have a really small clit, and only a little bit is visible. I knew how to touch it to get me off, but I have definitely had partners who I could tell were almost frantically searching for it! I'm pretty good now at guiding someone's hand and helping him find the right spot, but that is only because I had so many experiences where it just wasn't happening for me." Annette, thirty-two.

The best way to find out what works for you is to practice, either alone or with a partner. And remember, most things feel better when wetter. So if you aren't lubricated naturally, it is really good to use an artificial lube like Astroglide or KY jelly for clitoral stimulation.

The *Gräfenberg spot,* or *G-spot* ("discovered" by Ernst Gräfenberg, a German gynecologist), also known as the *urethral sponge,* is a small area of erectile tissue located on the front wall of the vagina between the *introitus* (opening of the vagina) and the cervix. It becomes engorged with blood during arousal and is particularly sensitive to stimulation—for some women, stimulation of the G-spot will lead to orgasms felt more internally than those felt from clitoral stimulation and female ejaculation (more about this later).

Female Sexual Response

A woman's sexual response can change from day to day and over the course of her life and be affected by any number of factors,

A WORD ABOUT FOREPLAY

The term *foreplay* was invented by people who write books on sex. Foreplay is what you are supposed to do to get a woman wet enough so the two of you can have intercourse . . . there is nothing caring about the underlying premise of foreplay: that women . . . need to be warmed up before they want to become sexual. Unfortunately, the concept of foreplay implies that tenderness is little more than a tollbooth on the big highway to intercourse. Nonsense. Tender kisses and caresses do not need to be trailed by intercourse to justify their importance or necessity. They are just as important as intercourse, if not more so.

If you can't get past the notion of foreplay, try to think of it as everything that's happened between you and your partner since the last time you had sex. How you treat each other with your clothes on has far more impact on what happens in bed than carefully planting kisses right before intercourse.

—From Paul Joannides, *Guide to Getting It On!*

such as sleep, hunger, menstrual cycle, emotion, mental health, physical health, and so on. Focusing primarily on orgasmic response shortchanges the entire sexual experience, which truly involves your body, senses, emotions, thoughts, memories, and relationship with others. This is not to say that orgasms don't deserve their place in the hall of fame, merely that we should give equal places of honor to all aspects of any experience. That said, it may be helpful to understand how that response works.

The female sexual response cycle is typically described in terms of four stages during which physiological and psychological changes occur: excitement/arousal, plateau, orgasm, and resolution. Excitement occurs when a woman is aroused by either psychological or physical stimulation. During this phase, women experience increased heart rate, respiration, muscle tension, and vaginal swelling and lubrication. Lubrication is a result of a process called *transudation,* in which vaginal walls "sweat" with a clear, slick fluid. If excitement is maintained, then a woman will enter the plateau stage, in which the breasts enlarge, the nipples become erect, the uterus drops to form something called the *seminal pool,* and the vagina lengthens.

The third stage, orgasm, involves a release of all the muscular tension that has been building during the previous two stages. Orgasm occurs when all the *myotonia,* or muscle tension, that occurs during sexual arousal is released. This results in very pleasurable feelings that may involve the whole body. During orgasm, heart rate increases, breathing quickens, blood pressure rate increases, and muscles throughout the body spasm and contract. The most intense spasms happen in the vagina, uterus, anus, and pelvic floor. Also during orgasm, chemicals called *endorphins* are released into the bloodstream. They cause pleasant sensations through the body, but they also make many women feel happy, tired, or warm. The combination of these sensations generally results in a very enjoyable feeling of release—lasting, surprisingly, for only seconds.

During the last stage, resolution, heart rate, swelling, breathing, basically everything returns to its original state. There is no set time that women should remain in each stage of the cycle because every woman is different. Some women move from excitement to orgasm quickly, some women who have multiple orgasms may move back and forth between plateau and orgasm many times before reaching the resolution stage, and some women may not reach orgasm at all.

Focusing on stages neglects the entire experience of female sexuality and perpetuates the belief that the "goal" of sexual encounters should be orgasm. So people tend to concentrate erroneously on the result rather than process. "Orgasm is often depicted in the media by thrashing moaning, gasping, writhing and fascinating gyrating behavior," write the authors of the insightful book *Sex Matters for Women*. ". . . It perpetuates the myth that a woman's orgasm is a spontaneously occurring event, happening as she is swept away in a consuming tidal wave of unbridled passion. Instead, we have come to know that a woman's orgasmic response is learned through experience, experimentation and self-awareness."

A woman can have an orgasm through stimulation of just her clitoris, just her vagina, or both, but most women have orgasms through stimulation of the clitoris. Vaginal, oral, or anal sex can result in an orgasm, as can any stimulation of the vulva. A partner can help a woman have an orgasm, and women can also masturbate to orgasm. Some women can even have an orgasm just by squeezing their thighs together or by fantasizing about sex.

Fewer than half of all women have orgasms during intercourse alone. During penetration, the clitoris does not usually get enough direct stimulation. So many women use fingers (their own or someone else's) to rub the clitoris, or may use a vibrator in conjunction with penetration.

Studies have shown that just as men have many erections throughout the night, women's vaginas go through regular patterns of lubrication while they are sleeping. When women have sexy dreams and become excited, it's common for their heart rate and blood pressure to spike, their nipples to get hard, and their breasts to enlarge. Blood flow increases to the genitals so that the clitoris swells and the vagina lubricates itself, producing wetness. Unlike men, women don't tend to leave any evidence in the morning that they have had an orgasm, so most don't even realize that it has occurred.

In general, there are three types of orgasms: clitoral, vaginal, and blended. During a clitoral orgasm, the vagina becomes longer; it causes a pocket to be formed beneath the uterus, sometimes called the seminal pool for its role in collecting semen during unprotected penile/vaginal sex. During a vaginal orgasm, the uterus drops lower and shortens the vagina. Stimulation of both the vagina and the clitoris can cause a blended orgasm, which is often characterized by breath holding. Each type of orgasm may feel slightly different from the other, but none is better—all are great.

A multiple orgasm typically involves a woman (or a man) experiencing several orgasms in one sexual session; they may happen one right after another, or they may come every few minutes. Having multiple orgasms is usually related to longer stimulation. While some of these orgasms may feel more or less intense, the intensity is not necessarily related to whether it is a woman's first, third, or fifth orgasm. According to the Web site femaleorgasm secrets.com, there are two kinds of multiple orgasms:

> **Sequential multiples**—a series of climaxes that come close together, usually from two to ten minutes apart. With sequential multiples there is an interruption in arousal before the first and second orgasm. A common scenario is oral sex climax followed by climax in penetrative vaginal intercourse.
> **Serial multiples**—orgasms that come one after the other, separated by seconds without interruption in arousal. Serial multiples occur during penetration when all the right spots are being stimulated (the clitoris, the G-spot, and so on).

"It's been my experience that no two orgasms are exactly alike," says Betty Dodson, sex educator extraordinaire and author of the classic book *Sex for One*. "The most common type is the 'tension orgasm,' where all the muscles tighten up until there's an explosion. Then it's all over. I call that one a 'maintenance orgasm,' kind of like my childhood orgasms when I held my breath and didn't move my body and came as fast as I could so no one would catch me masturbating. As a teenager, I did 'sleeping beauty orgasms' with complete relaxation. I certainly didn't want to act sexy, so there was no heavy breathing and no humping because that would have damaged my 'good girl' image. So we'd kiss and my boyfriend would fondle my clitoris while I remained passive and beautiful until all of a sudden—the orgasm would come and get me. My attitude was, 'I'm not responsible, I didn't do anything, my body did that.' Eventually I got into a combination of tension and relaxation that I call the 'rock-and-roll orgasm.' That's how an athlete uses her body: Your muscles are tense and then you let them go, then they tense up again and you let them go, and it's rhythmic. That's the whole idea of fucking, moving rhythmically and breathing. So I'm definitely into the rock-and-roll orgasm, but I whip out those little tension orgasms when the pressure is on. As far as I'm concerned, I don't have the patience to do the sleeping beauty or the total relaxation orgasm anymore: Last time I tried, I just went to sleep. But I always say, 'Whatever gets you off, go for it.'"

About 10 percent of women ejaculate when they orgasm, and they don't necessarily understand what is happening when they do. In fact, women often report that they thought they were urinating when they first ejaculated. Ejaculation in both men and women involves the release of fluid from the urethra. But female ejaculate is not urine. The liquid that makes up ejaculate actually is a lot more like male ejaculate.

Cunning Linguistics

Cunnilingus, derived from the Latin cunnus (vulva) and lingere (to lick), literally means "licking vulva." But oral sex is not just about licking—sucking, stroking, blowing air, humming, and nibbling are some of the many ways of pleasuring the vulva orally.

Every woman enjoys different techniques, ways of being touched, amount of time spent, and types of pressure for oral sex. The only way to know is to ask, either before you begin or while you're trying to please. Some vulvas enjoy a firmer, more direct tongue penetration, while others prefer an indirect sucking on the lips and clitoral hood. Don't forget that the vulva is

OOOORG&SMMMS

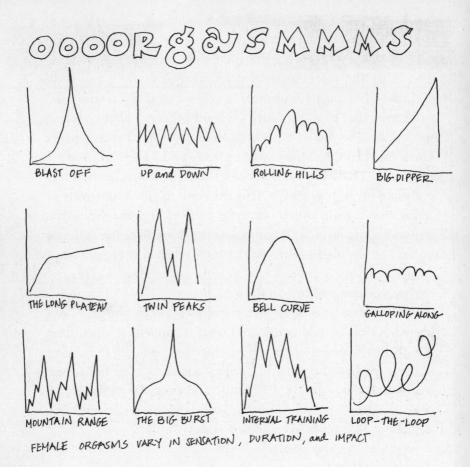

BLAST OFF UP and DOWN ROLLING HILLS BIG DIPPER

THE LONG PLATEAU TWIN PEAKS BELL CURVE GALLOPING ALONG

MOUNTAIN RANGE THE BIG BURST INTERVAL TRAINING LOOP-THE-LOOP

FEMALE ORGASMS VARY IN SENSATION, DURATION, and IMPACT

more than the clitoris (and the clitoris itself has many dimensions), so explore inner thighs, outer and inner lips, and the perineum as well. What someone enjoys may change over the course of one evening as the session goes on. Pay attention to your partner's body and verbal language as an indicator of how it's going. An "ouch" means stop and ask!

Speaking of the clitoris, some women find direct touching of the clitoral tip to be too intense or uncomfortable. Sucking or licking over the hood or to the side of the clitoris may feel better. Some women enjoy a particular spot and, once you've found it, prefer that you stay there (maybe forever). Keep in mind that as arousal grows, a woman may want you to speed up or slow down, change the amount of pressure you're applying, and/or shift the location of your licking or sucking or nibbling. You may want to try stopping for a few seconds every once in a while to generate buildup of excitement and anticipation.

Using a mouth and tongue, you can create a variety of pleasurable sensations for the vulva. Try French-kissing the vulva passionately as you would a mouth. The tongue itself can be used in a variety of ways. The tip of the tongue can be used to probe, prod, and penetrate. The flat part of the tongue can lick, stroke, and envelop. You can draw circles, triangles, or the letter Z or M, or you can write the entire alphabet (or a secret message for her to decode) with your tongue. A lubricated tongue that is covered with saliva works best, so if you are prone to dry mouth, make sure you have a glass of water or other form of lubricant handy.

Depending upon what position you are in for this delicious activity, you may or may not have a free hand. If you do, using your free hand to press or rub her breasts/nipples or the mons pubis in a circular motion may intensify the pleasure. Inserting one, two, three, or more fingers into her vagina or anus can make the oral experience intensely pleasurable.

A woman may gyrate her hips, stay perfectly still, or even buck up and down during oral sex, so be prepared for possible motion. Here are more tips for oral pleasuring, adapted from the *Guide to Getting It On!*:

- **The Hoover Maneuver. Experiment by puckering your lips around the clitoris and sucking in lightly. You can then push the clitoris in and out of your mouth either with your tongue or by reversing the suction rhythmically.**

- Butt'er Up. Place pillows under the buttocks for easier access to the vulva and to create tension in her pelvis and inner thighs.
- Weather Report. To heat things up, blow warm, moist air through the front panel of her underwear or sip a warm beverage before kissing the vulva. Never blow air directly into the vagina. To cool things off, place a small ice cube in her vagina or run it around the edges of her vulva.

Here are some other thoughts about oral sex:

"I am now seventy-one years of age and a widower. I find widows will still let me have it, especially because I know how to give them a good blow job. Many women of my age have never had that before. Once you give it to them, they want it all the time." Arthur, seventy-one.

"I am especially fond of long pussy lips and excited ones that get fat when horny. . . . I also love large clits. . . . When a woman is very horny and her clit is filled with blood, it is so sensitive and I just love to touch it with my tongue and hold it there. You can feel it pulse and sometimes make a woman come just holding it there softly." Carlos, thirty-eight.

"My girlfriend does this amazing thing when I'm straddling her face and she's eating me out. She takes a Pocket Rocket [a small vibrator] and holds it on top of my clit while she flicks her tongue underneath. It sends me through the roof." Jannah, forty-three.

Safer Oral Sex

Cunnilingus can put you at risk for the following sexually transmitted infections: herpes, gonorrhea, human papillomavirus, the virus that causes genital warts, and HIV. Many people don't know that a cold sore is herpes (herpes simplex) and that if you have a cold sore on your lip or nose and perform oral sex, you can transmit that herpes to her vulva or anus. Having oral sex during a woman's period is riskier for HIV transmission than having it at other times of the month.

For safer cunnilingus, use a dental dam (see illustration on page 110) or plastic wrap to cover the vulva before putting your mouth on it. A dental dam is a large, thin square of latex that provides a barrier between mouth and vulva or mouth and anus. If you find dams too small, you can also use run-of-the-mill plastic wrap for the same purpose. No studies have yet shown the effectiveness of plastic wrap as a barrier to viruses and bacteria, but many health educators believe it is effective—it's at least much safer than going without! Plastic wrap is cheaper than purchased latex barriers, and you can use as much as you want or need. Never reuse a dental dam or plastic wrap, and be careful that you don't inadvertently reverse the barrier and expose yourself and your partner to possible infection. Add lubricant to the lickee's side to help increase sensation.

Entering Vagina Land

*Y*ou can enter V-land with many items, including fingers, fists, toes, dildos, vibrators (or other sex toys), or a penis. *Never* penetrate a vagina with an open bottle, as it can create dangerous suction. Being sexually aroused and lubricated (whether it's your own or added lube) can make penetration more comfortable. The general rule is to go slowly and stop if there is any pain. It may take a number of sessions before you are able to have comfortable vaginal intercourse, particularly if you have never been penetrated, if you haven't been penetrated in a long time, or if you have had unpleasant or violent penetrative encounters. If you consistently experience painful penetration, please consult a medical provider to ascertain if a physical condition is causing the discomfort. Some women enjoy being

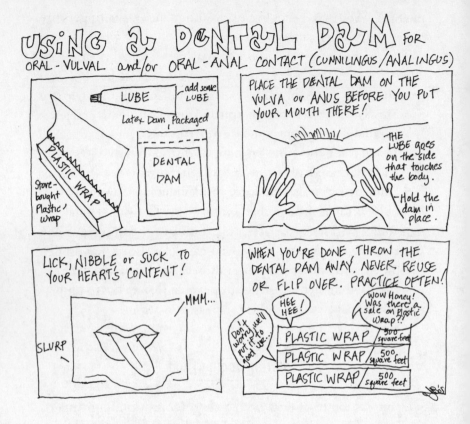

penetrated, while others prefer to stick with clitoral stimulation and other "outercourse" activities.

Following are brief descriptions of a few ways to penetratively pleasure a vagina.

Hand in the Bush

One, two, three, four, or more fingers can be used to pleasure the vagina. Playing with the vulva (teasing the lips with your fingertips, exploring all the nooks and crannies) before entering may be preferable for some women. It will help arousal and facilitate lubrication (although I always recommend adding lube;

one can never have enough lubricant!). Once your fingers are inside the vaginal canal, you have many options. Here are some favorites:

- Gently wiggle your fingers, creating a vibrator effect.
- Slowly make circles around the perimeter of the vaginal canal about a quarter-inch inside.
- Inside the vagina is the G-spot, which is located about an inch or so inside the vaginal opening on the anterior (front) wall. Hook your fingers up toward her belly button and feel for a smooth part of the vaginal wall. This will be the G-spot. Stimulate it by pressing, rubbing, or tickling it.
- Thrust your fingers in and out of the vagina, varying the rhythm and inserting them more slowly than you withdraw them.
- Insert one lubricated finger into her anus while keeping the others in her vagina. Do *not* reinsert the anus finger back into the vagina.
- If you have inserted two fingers, simulate a "walking" motion so that as one moves forward, the other moves back. You can speed up or slow down this motion.

For safer fingering, wear a latex or polyurethane glove and apply a water-based lubricant to both the glove and her vagina.

Phallic Phun

Whether using a penis, a vibrator, or a dildo, take the time to consider a woman's degree of readiness for phallic penetration. Inserting a penis or other object into a dry, unwelcoming vagina will at best be uncomfortable and at worst be painful. Asking if she is ready or asking her to let you know when she is ready is one great way to take the guesswork out of this.

Another is to let her guide the penis or object inside (also ensuring a smoother entry; it's easy to miss when you're in the moment) rather than trying to put it inside when you think it's the right time for you.

Different women have different preferences (surprise!) for the way they like to be entered. Some prefer teasing around the vulva (try rubbing up and down, enveloped by her lips) before entering, some prefer a slow inching in, some like a long, deep first thrust. These preferences can change depending upon many factors, including your emotional connections, how close she is to orgasm, what position you're in (standing, sitting, on your knees; on the top, bottom, or side; legs bent, open, or close together), or the length of her vagina in relation to the length of the penis, dildo, or vibrator.

Alternating shallow and deep thrusts can be fun, especially since (according to Paul Joannides) "shallow thrusting encourages the snuggest part of the vagina to wrap around the most sensitive part of the penis . . . [It] also allows the ridge around the head of the penis to stimulate this sensitive part of the vagina . . . Deep thrusting can help to position his pubic bone in direct contact with her clitoral area . . . [and] may allow the penis to pull on the inner lips for a longer period of time, providing more stimulation to the clitoral area." Sounds like a win-win situation to me.

Some women don't like thrusting at all, preferring a slow rocking or a circular, grinding motion with the penis or other object staying inside. Play with the rhythm, tempo, beat . . . create your own original music.

Safer Penetration

Unprotected penile-vaginal penetration can put you at risk for any number of sexually transmitted infections, including HIV, herpes, genital warts, gonorrhea, syphilis, hepatitis B, parasites (such as crabs), and chlamydia. Correctly and consistently using a latex or polyurethane condom (including the Female Condom) can greatly reduce the risk of infection and unintended pregnancy. For more information about sexually transmitted infections, go to the American Social Health Association's excellent Web site at www.ashastd.org

For instructions on the correct use of condoms, see chapter 7, "A Penile Pilgrimage."

What did you learn in this chapter?

_____

_____

What did you read that surprised you?

_____

_____

What would you like to learn more about?

_____

_____

Something I learned about vulvas and vaginas from reading this chapter is:

_____

_____

WORKSHEET: FOR THOSE
WITH VULVAS AND VAGINAS

For many women, their genitals are a bit of a mystery. Unlike men, women may have to work a bit harder to find theirs. The following worksheet will help you figure out how you feel about your vulva and vagina.

Before reading this chapter, did you know the difference between your vulva and your vagina?

Yes _____   No _____   Don't Know _____

If yes, how did you learn the difference?

_____

_____

What do you call your vulva? _____

What term do you use when you are with a sexual
partner? _____

What do you call it when you are at the doctor's
office? _____

Have you ever looked at your vulva in the mirror? If not, why
not? If so, what were your thoughts about it the first time you
saw it?

_____

_____

I think my vulva is:
    Pretty   ❑
    Normal   ❑
    Ugly   ❑
    Cute   ❑
    Weird   ❑
    Sexy   ❑
    Other: _____

My favorite part(s) of my vulva (check all that apply):

Outer labia ❏

Clitoris ❏

Public hair ❏

The whole deal! ❏

Other: _____

If there was one thing I could change about my vulva, it would be:

_____

My vulva tastes like: _____

My vulva smells like: _____

My vulva looks like: _____

Partners have given me this compliment(s) about my vulva:

_____

Partners have given me this compliment(s) about my vagina:

_____

My vulva enjoys the following:

_____

_____

My vagina enjoys the following:

_____

_____

IT'S NOT THE SIZE OF THE SHIP

Some women have bigger vaginas, some women have smaller. Most people agree it is not the size of someone's vagina that makes a sexual experience pleasurable. But a woman might want to strengthen her vaginal muscles. Strengthening these muscles can actually help a woman's sexual response, and her partner may also experience different sensations if she works these muscles during clitoral stimulation and vaginal penetration. It can also help with urinary continence. Vagina exercises are called Kegels. These exercises involve strengthening the *pubococcygeal* (PC) muscle. You can find the PC muscle by stopping the stream of urine when you are peeing. The muscle that you use to do this is the PC muscle. Check out the following guide for more info about Kegels.

Kegels 101
- Contract your PC muscle.
- Hold for a count of five.
- Relax your PC muscle.
- Repeat ten times, eight to ten times a day.

Kegels 102
- Slow Kegels: Tighten your PC muscle and hold for a slow count of three. Relax and repeat ten times.
- Fast Kegels: Tighten and relax the PC muscle as rapidly as you can for about ten seconds.
- Fluttering: Quickly tighten and release your PC muscle in a fluttering movement for ten seconds. Relax for ten seconds and repeat.

Equipment
You can buy a Kegel barbell to help in your exercises. These are specially designed medical devices, but many women-run sex toy shops or Web sites sell them as well.

Chapter 7

A PENILE PILGRIMAGE

What You Need to Know About Male Genitals

* * *

Testy-esty-esticles
Scrotie-otie-otium
Ballie-awlie-awlials
Go-nads, go!
—Male genital cheer
attributed to Elliot Austin

*W*hether you're an owner or a visitor to the land of penises, it's helpful to know a few key phallus facts to make the journey more "phantastic."

As opposed to women, who often do not know what their vulvas or vaginas look like, men are usually intimately acquainted with their penis and testicles. They touch them first thing in the morning and last thing at night, often sleeping with their hand resting gently on their genitals for protection. The average male urinates between five and seven times a day, which requires pulling out, holding, aiming, shaking, and tucking in the penis. But that doesn't mean that men know everything there is to know about a part of the body that probably has more nicknames than any other.

Penises come in a wide variety of shapes, sizes, and colors. Some penises are long and lean, others are short and thick; some men have hair on their penis, whiles others have smooth or wrinkly bare skin. It's normal for the skin on the penis to have *papules*, or little bumps. Some penises have heads that are partially covered with foreskin, some have heads totally covered with foreskin, and others have no foreskin at all.

What Do You Call It?

anteater	dong	narmer	rod	unit
bat n balls	firehose	noodle	sausage	wang
battery	goshu	ock	schlong	weenie
big boy	hot dog	one-eyed snake	shaft	wee-wee
big papa	jimmy	papi	shmuck	whistle
bologna	Johnson	pecker	shotgun	wiener
bornk	joystick	pedro	snake	willy
bratwurst	king cobra	pee-pee	spikey	woody
cannon	liquid snake	pencil	stick	worm
chinpoko	lollypop	peter	switch	yogurt slinger
cobra	Long John	pickle	thing	
cock	magnum	pipe	thingy	
Colt 45	manhood	pisspump	tool	
deez	meat	piss station	Tootsie-Roll	
dick	microphone	prick	trigger	
dingaling	mini me	punga	trousersnake	
dink	missile	putz	tweeter	

—From Rutgers University human sexuality class

Size Matters

$\mathcal{I}$'m not going to pretend that people never prefer larger or smaller penises. Preference is just part of human nature. However, few men or women list penis size as a crucial element of what makes someone a sexy or desirable sex partner. Unfortunately, we live in a "supersize it" society. Bigger is often assumed to be better. When it comes to penis size, this just isn't the case.

A lot of men worry that their penis is not going to be big enough to please a partner. But before someone decides to throw in the towel because he doesn't look like Dirk Diggler, consider the following:

- Most men do not look like porn stars! The average size of a soft penis is about 3.25 to 4.25 inches. For around 85 percent of men, the average length of a hard penis is 5 to 7 inches, and the average circumference is 4.9 inches around.
- The size of a man's penis when it is flaccid has nothing to do with how big it will become when erect. In fact, smaller flaccid penises tend to grow more when they become erect than do penises that are larger when soft.
- Men are notoriously bad at estimating their own penis size. In one study, men who initially claimed to be ten or more inches long turned out, on actual measuring, to be considerably smaller.

Some men are worried that they won't be able to please someone sexually if they don't have a huge penis. That's just not true. In fact, most people agree that being above average in the sack has little to do with whether a man's penis is above average in length.

Other men worry that their penis is too large for comfortable sex play, both vaginal and anal. Unlike the penis, the vagina is a muscle that can expand and contract—enough to let a baby pass through—and as we all know, the penis is nowhere near as large as a baby. Even so, it helps to know a bit about how female sexual response actually works. When a woman becomes sexually aroused, her vagina elongates and lubricates, but this doesn't necessarily happen immediately. Women may need varying amounts and types of stimulation before they are ready for vaginal penetration. For some women, this may mean deep kissing; for others, it means oral sex. But some women still won't get that wet even if they are totally turned on, owing to everything from age to medication to diet.

Unlike the vagina, the anus never produces enough natural lubrication for comfortable sex play. The good news is that, like the vagina, the anus can expand to accommodate a penis or other object. Still, for both vaginal and anal sex, it is really important to go slowly and listen to your partner. If something hurts, don't do it! For a lot of people, gentle penetration with a finger or dildo can help facilitate later penile penetration. Big penis or small, there are ways to make sex play more pleasurable. That's why artificial lube was invented—I recommend making it an integral part of your sex play repertoire (see "Lubricants," page 216).

Penises come not only in different sizes, but in different shapes. A curved penis is fairly common. Some men are born with curved penises, and others are curved because of a buildup of scar tissue inside the shaft that may have been caused by minor trauma to the shaft during erection or as a complication of circumcision. This scar tissue can pull the entire shaft to curve to the side or in a downward direction. Men with a curvature of the penis can usually still have intercourse and ejaculate. If a man's curvature is so severe that it is hindering his sexual experiences, he may want to opt for a medical intervention.

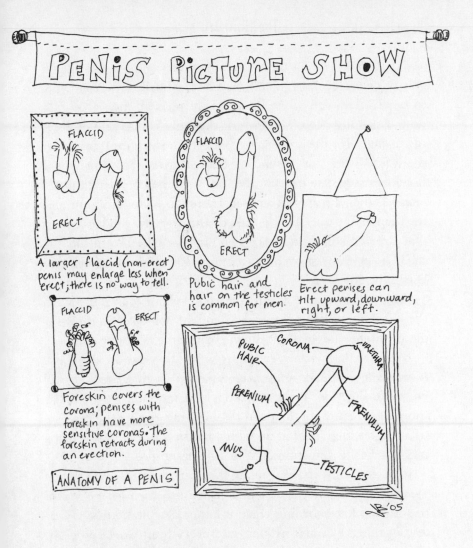

PENIS PICTURE SHOW

A larger flaccid (non-erect) penis may enlarge less when erect; there is no way to tell.

Pubic hair and hair on the testicles is common for men.

Erect penises can tilt upward, downward, right, or left.

Foreskin covers the corona; penises with foreskin have more sensitive coronas. The foreskin retracts during an erection.

ANATOMY OF A PENIS

Care and Feeding of a Penis

*Y*our sweaty genitals need their daily dose of soap and water, too. If you have a penis with foreskin, it is important to pull back the foreskin and wash the head of the penis. The taste of a penis can be arousing, but for most people the taste of *smegma* is not.

The Hard Truth

*A*n erection means that a penis has gotten stiffer and bigger. A man's penis becomes erect when he is sexually aroused, owing to excitement, and when he is deeply relaxed, such as during deep, dreaming sleep. The shaft of the penis is made up of erectile tissue called the *corpora cavernosa*, which runs from just under the *glans* all the way down the shaft. Normally, a penis is in a flaccid or soft state because the spaces in the erectile tissue are empty. When a man gets aroused, more blood flows into his penis than flows out. This is called *vasocongestion,* and it occurs when the erectile tissue relaxes enough for blood to fill the tissue. The penis must swell to accommodate all this new blood— hence the erection.

Erect penises can curve to the right or left (curving toward the left is about five times more frequent) and vary in their angle, pointing straight ahead, down, or optimistically upward.

Men can have many erections while they are in rapid eye movement sleep, and they may wake up to find they are still erect. An erection in the morning, as at any time, is caused by more blood entering the penis than leaving, not by the pressure of a full bladder. Waking up with a hard-on can be a sign that a man has healthy erections, not that he has to pee.

It is not only the mornings that can produce unexpected erections. Spontaneous erections happen to men for no sexual reason, and like morning erections, they are the body's way of testing things out and making sure everything works properly. They can pop up at the most surprising and often inopportune times—during that big presentation or five minutes into first meeting the in-laws.

A lot of men get really freaked out by these hard-ons. But here are a few things to know that may calm you down. You are not a big pervert if you find yourself with an erection halfway through *Dumbo*. What can you do about this ill-timed bulge?

Every man has to find his own trick. Count backward from one hundred. Do math problems in your head. Conjugate French verbs. Think about your declining stock portfolio. Remember how sad you felt when ET was being dissected by scary scientists and Elliott couldn't get inside to help. In any case, erections come and go, and often just ignoring the little guy will make him return to his comfortably flaccid state.

But what if this is a regular problem or you have an erection that just won't go away? In rare cases, a man may have what is called a *priapism*. A priapism is a prolonged and painful erection that can last from several hours up to a few days. The priapismic erection is not associated with sexual thoughts or sexual activity. What happens is that blood flows into the penis but is unable to drain as it would normally. Most priapisms are due to particular medications or specific medical conditions. It is advisable to seek treatment for an erection that has gone on for more than four to six hours. Failing to do so can result in the creation of scar tissue in the penis, which can lead to impotence.

Men of any age can have difficulties obtaining or maintaining an erection. The advent of Viagra has brought the issue of erectile dysfunction to the public consciousness, but this consciousness has excluded younger men who might be affected. Erectile dysfunction can happen for a million reasons. Age, disease, and medication are common causes, but alcohol or other drug use, fear, depression, exhaustion, and uncertainty about a partner can also contribute. Some men report that if they are afraid of causing a pregnancy or contracting a sexually transmitted infection, it is difficult for them to become hard. It is fairly common and normal for erections to vary even throughout one sexual encounter. Penises become harder and softer at different times during sex play. Just be aware of these fluctuations, so that a condom doesn't slip off when your erection is getting a little softer.

A lot of young men experience premature ejaculation when

they first become sexually active owing to excitement, change of sensation, and years of masturbating hurriedly to come quickly so that they don't get caught in the bathroom. But young men don't have the market cornered—just ask someone who has had this happen to him at the ripe old age of twenty-five or thirty-five or forty-five. Early ejaculation is normal and can happen because of inexperience or periods of abstinence, nervousness, drug or alcohol use, and the ever popular "just because."

The amount of time it takes for a man to get an erection af-ter ejaculating is called the *refractory period*. A young man may have a refractory period of a few seconds, while an older man might have a refractory period that lasts an entire day. If your partner has a long refractory period, there are many other ways he can be sexual that do not focus on the penis. He can still en-joy physical touch and contact. Kissing, body rubbing, role-play, anal play, and pleasuring a partner are all activities that a man can do whether he has an erection or not.

Color Me Blue?

"When I was fourteen I wouldn't give my boyfriend a hand job, and he spent weeks complaining to me and everyone else we knew about his ex-cruciating blue balls. I am twenty-seven now, and I have never met an-other guy who suffered from blue balls. I was always kind of skeptical." Maya, twenty-seven.

"I was thirteen years old when I had my first case of blue balls. I was over at my girlfriend's house, and we were alone in her bedroom. I decided to go ahead with a little bit of sexual experimentation, some-thing I had never done before—I stuck the pointer finger of my right hand deep inside her moist, beautifully textured vagina. The results were probably very small for her, but I was amazed—oh my God, this is the

best thing that has ever happened to my finger, not to mention my pecker—and I got the biggest boner ever.

"A short while after that, I skateboarded home with a tent in my pants and a grin the size of a mountain. When I got home I disguised my tent as best I could by tucking my boner up into the elastic of my underwear. Both my parents were in the kitchen making dinner, and after a quick hello I dashed to the living room to watch a bit of TV.

"Note: When I was about ten years old, I suffered from testicle torsion—one of 'em twisted till it wouldn't twist anymore. It righted itself very quickly, but the doctors suggested surgery to prevent it from happening again. I got the surgery when I was twelve.

"So I'm watching TV and finding it hard to get comfortable. Something is wrong, something is desperately wrong. I stroll/waddle into the kitchen. 'Hey, Pop, can I show you something in the living room?' I say. 'Sure,' he replies. We walk toward the living room, and along the way I grab his arm and pull him into the bathroom. 'Dad, my balls, man, my balls,' I strain. 'What? What are you talking about?' my father replies with a voice of concern. 'Don't tell Mom, but we need to go to emergency, I think I twisted my testicle again. I don't want Mom to worry,' I say. 'Okay, I'll get dressed, and we can go,' he says.

"A few moments later, he comes down the stairs and walks up to me. What seemed to be out of the blue, he asks, 'Did you fool around with a girl today?' A bit embarrassed, I reply, 'Yes.' 'Did you, you know, ejaculate?' He stumbles over his words a bit. 'No,' I respond.

"And just when I thought the awkwardness might be over, a look of relief comes over his face and he says, 'Okay, you have blue balls'— and this is the part that I always remember in slow motion—'go upstairs and jerk off.' My father just told me to masturbate. The one thing that I have been so successful in hiding for several years, my father just told me to do. With an edge of frustration, confusion, and embarrassment all wrapped up into a nice, miserable package, I shout, 'What?' 'You'll feel better,' he replies. 'Do you need any material?' " Michael, thirty-two.

Pleasurable Moments for Penises

Insert Penis, Please

Penises thrive in a warm, wet environment (think tropical rain forest). They derive pleasure from being immersed in a saliva-filled mouth, embraced by a hand saturated with lotion, inserted into a moist vaginal canal, or submerged in a well-lubricated anus. They also enjoy being stroked, touched, kissed, and licked. The following penis "hot spots" are sure to please:

- Go for the glans! The head of the penis (or *glans*) is one of the most sensitive parts. Someone who is uncircumcised and has a foreskin will usually have a more sensitive glans than someone who is circumcised.
- My corona! The *corona* is the anatomically correct name for the ridge that is at the bottom of the head, another penis hot spot. Many men enjoy the running of a finger or tongue around the corona. In men who are uncircumcised, the corona may not be completely visible until or even during erection, but it's still a pleasure zone for most men.
- Fren-ul-yum! The *frenulum* is on the underside of the corona. It's a little y-shaped membrane on the top of the shaft of the penis, just under the head. On uncircumcised men, it's what attaches the foreskin to the shaft of the penis. On circumcised men, it is a highly sensitive small ridge of skin or scar tissue. Many men are able to ejaculate just by continued stimulation of this hot spot with fingers or a tongue.
- Perin-e-yum! The *perineum,* aka the male G-spot, is the area that runs from the bottom of the testicles (where they attach to the body) to the anus. This section of

skin is incredibly sensitive, and many men like to have it caressed, tongued, or otherwise stroked with the tips of fingers, knuckles, or a vibrator during sex play. You can also internally massage the perineum by inserting a gloved or lubricated finger or sex toy into the anus (for more on this, see page 219, "Backdoor Basics").

Down Below

Many, many books are written on the topic of ways to pleasure a penis orally. Whether authored by gay, straight, or bisexual men who have penises or by those who enjoy penises, the ultimate premise of these books is that for most men, oral sex, also referred to as *fellatio,* rules. Joseph, forty-six, says, "There is nothing like the feeling of having my dick immersed in a warm, wet mouth." "It's great when I can just lie back and relax and be serviced by my woman," says Tyrone, twenty-nine.

All of these books offer time-tested techniques for titillating, teasing, and tonguing a penis. Keep in mind that no one method works for everyone every time (we are not machines, we are human beings), so if what you're doing isn't rocking his world at that moment, don't despair. Try another technique or consider that maybe he's just not that into it at that time because of stress, not feeling well, or other stuff that's going on (not necessarily anything to do with you).

Following is a description of the basic oral sex technique from *Sex Tips for Straight Women from a Gay Man* by Dan Anderson (Regan Books, 1997). My personal comments are in brackets:

If you're starting out with Mr. Softee [that's a non-erect penis], you should have no trouble putting the whole thing in your mouth while you gently suck and lick. Don't start moving your mouth up and down until he's at least semierect. Make a ring around the base of the shaft with your hand, which will help him grow harder quicker. Take a sip of water [always a good idea to keep some water nearby in case of dry mouth]. . . . Put both hands into an "L" position [or use one hand to form a ring around the shaft] around the base of his shaft. Lick the whole tip, and then use your tongue to lick up and down the sides. Now it should be slick enough to slide into your mouth easily. Covering your teeth with your lips, and keeping your mouth taut, glide the head inside and lick the sensitive spot underneath with both the tip and the flat part of your tongue—like what you would use on . . . [an] ice cream cone. Still covering your teeth and maintaining your pressure, proceed down the shaft as far as you can go in one fell swoop [very few people can put the entire penis in their mouth; go down as far as you can]. . . . Pull your mouth back up the entire length of the shaft right over the ridge of the tip. He'll love the sensation of your lips popping over this ridge [it's that glans/corona thing]. Take it out of your mouth for a second, then go right back down. This will give you a chance to breathe. Continue the full up-and-down motion at a sensual, slow pace . . . usually after about two or three minutes [please don't time it, just trust your instincts on when to start the next part] it's time to start using your hand. With [one] hand, make a ring with your thumb and forefinger and follow the movement of your lips up and down [this serves as a "mouth extender" that enables you to be in control of how much of the penis is going into your mouth, which reduces the chances of gagging]. One hand [can] remain at the base of the penis to keep it in place [or use it to play gently with his testicles]. Maintain a slow pace. Stopping, starting, stopping, and starting again may make for a bigger, better, and much more powerful orgasm [not true for everyone; sometimes stopping is distracting—you'll just have to ask] . . . go into a fast ring technique–mouth combo [you can add a twist of your hand to the up-and-down motion for variety]. . . . When's he's ready to let rip, move your head out of the way or prepare to swallow. Keep stroking with your hand till it's over [when no more cum is coming].

Most other oral sex techniques are a takeoff on this basic methodology: different hand or mouth positions, changing speed or direction or pressure, sucking, humming, or making other noises, putting various substances in your mouth like mouthwash or a mint for a fresh, cool, tingly feeling, ice cubes for a stunning climate change, or whipped cream for soft, blanketlike warmth. Here are some other fellatio tips:

- **Be handy. Use your free hand to lightly scratch his inner thighs, tease his pubic hair, play with his testicles (gently, unless he asks for them to be squeezed more forcefully), or stroke his perineum.***
- **French-kiss the penis. Imagine that you're kissing the penis in the way that you would explore a mouth with your tongue. Keep your tongue moving, and vary the way in which you use it: Flick the tip of your tongue around the glans, use the wide part of your tongue to lick the corona, wiggle your tongue down the shaft, use the underside of your tongue on the frenulum—the possibilities are endless.**

---

* Adapted from Lou Paget's *How to Be a Great Lover* (Random House, 1999).

- Try "the Big W."* Starting with your tongue burrowed into the area where his leg attaches to his groin, move your tongue (as if you're writing with it) in the shape of a large W, going down one side of the scrotum, up between his balls, and finishing the stroke on the other side of the scrotum. Reverse and repeat as needed.
- Nibbles and bits. Use your teeth to nibble the shaft of the penis—kind of like you're eating an ear of corn, bite gently around the glans, use your teeth to create a new sensation when going up and down the shaft, or chomp on his pubic hair or his inner thighs.
- Got rhythm? In some way, good fellatio is all about finding your rhythm, that combination of up and down, slow and fast, hard and soft, that works for each person. If there's music playing in the background, you can use that to help guide you as you get going (up 2-3-4, down 6-7-8). Get to know your partner's body and the signs that he's about to come (the penis gets incredibly hard or he starts to moan), and work with him to figure out the rhythm that will rock his world.

Spit, Swallow, or Towel?

Let's take a minute to talk about what actually comes out when a man ejaculates. *Ejaculate,* also called *cum, semen,* or *jizz,* is the fluid that is released from the urethra of the penis after sexual stimulation. Ejaculate is made up of a number of different fluids that are contributed by different parts of the male reproductive system. The one we hear most about is sperm. Sperm are the little swimmers that are made in the testicles and can cause a pregnancy—but sperm make up only a part of the

---

* Adapted from Lou Paget's *How to Be a Great Lover* (Random House, 1999).

ejaculate. After leaving the testicles, sperm pick up various fluids on their journey to release. Most crucial is fluid from the erectile duct and prostate. Prostatic fluid contributes a lot of bulk to ejaculate. It is a burst of fluid from the prostate that forces ejaculate out of the penis. This can actually happen at— hold on to your condoms—up to sixty miles an hour! Semen can be whitish, yellowish, opaque, or translucent in color. It can be thick or thin and just like peanut butter, smooth or chunky in texture. There is a lot of variety in what makes up healthy ejaculate.

There's no universal agreement on spitting versus swallowing versus not coming in the mouth and oral sex. Personal preference rules. However, swallowing and spitting are more risky for sexually transmitted infections. Some people enjoy it when their partner comes on their chest (also called a *pearl necklace*), on their stomach, or on other body parts. Keeping a towel handy for cleaning up can help you avoid the "I must get up now and get something to wipe that sticky stuff from your hair" moment. Wet semen is still potent and can cause pregnancy (if it gets into the vagina) and/or transmit infection.

Safer Oral Sex for a Penis

Using a condom for oral sex can reduce your risk of transmitting or receiving such sexually transmitted infections as HIV, gonorrhea, hepatitis B, and herpes (so if you have a cold sore on your mouth, which is herpes, be extra careful). Condoms come in a variety of flavors, and even the boring normal-tasting ones can be jazzed up with flavored lubricant or non-oil-containing tasty treats like jelly or yogurt. For those with tongue dexterity (like my talented friend who can tie a knot in a cherry stem using only her tongue), putting on a condom with your mouth can provide an enticing incentive for safer sex. Following is one method for doing this. Feel free to practice first on a dildo, a banana, or a cucumber.

- Put a clear, water-based lubricant on your lips. You can either apply the lube to your lips yourself or have your partner do it for you.

- Remove a condom from its package and make sure it is in the correct position for unrolling. If you hold the reservoir tip (the nipplelike part at the top) between your thumb and forefinger and the condom looks like a hat with a brim, it is in the correct position.

- Put a tiny bit of water-based lubricant in the reservoir tip of the condom so that the condom will slide gently over the penis, giving your partner more sensation.

- Pucker up as if you were going to kiss someone, but keep your lips slightly apart. Put the condom in your mouth using a slight sucking motion to keep it in place. The rim of the "hat" should be outside your lips.

- Hold the shaft of the penis in one hand and move your mouth to the top of the head of the penis. Place the rim of the condom on the head of the penis, but keep the rest of the condom in your mouth and push the rim down gently with your tongue to remove any air bubbles.

- Wrap your lips over your teeth and gently but firmly unroll the condom onto the shaft of the penis in one smooth motion. Depending upon your comfort level, you may not be able to go all the way down to the bottom of the shaft. In that case, use your fingers (making a circle with your thumb and forefinger around the condom) to unroll the rest.

Hand Jobs

Giving a hand job is, basically, masturbating someone else. The best way to learn what someone likes is to ask him how he masturbates. From that basic knowledge, you can proceed with his "time-tested technique" or work to change different elements in hand motion, rhythm and tempo, and position (there are certain positions and techniques that he can't do to his own penis, which gives you an advantage with originality and uniqueness). Please keep lubricant "handy" for these adventures.

The following stories emphasize the importance of using lubricant:

"So, there I was, in college, dating this guy from a fraternity. It's my first time touching a penis, and I'm just rubbing away. He is grimacing, in ecstasy, so I thought. After a while he says, gritting his teeth, 'Could . . . you . . . please . . . not . . . rub . . . so . . . hard!' I was so embarrassed. I didn't know penises were so sensitive. I think I had taken off a layer of his skin. After his penis healed, about a week later, he showed me how to do it." Katie, fifty-two.

"I didn't actually hook up with a girl until I was in my twenties, but I had been masturbating for a long time, so I knew what I liked. And what I liked was hand cream. The first girl I was with was not aware of this and started wrenching at my dick in this really jerky way. The whole time I wanted to just open my drawer and hand her the cream, but I was worried that she would think I didn't want to hook up with her, so I just suffered silently and prayed that I would come soon!" Lebron, twenty-nine.

Entering Through the Back Door

Many men enjoy anal play whether they are gay, straight, bisexual, or questioning their sexual orientation. The anus is a part of the body, and enjoying anal stimulation is not an indication of sexual orientation. One of the reasons people like anal stimulation is that the anus has a lot of nerve endings that can feel really good when touched. Many men believe that it is not manly to be penetrated. They are taught that women are penetrated and men do the penetrating. But this rigid definition of gender roles is both inaccurate and unfortunate, as it limits sexual exploration and potential pleasure.

Both men and women can enjoy the sensation of fullness that

comes from anal play, and a lot of men can experience prostate stimulation through the anus. Stimulation of this gland can be pleasurable in and of itself, or it can intensify a man's orgasm. Some men can even orgasm from prostate stimulation alone, whether or not their penis is being stimulated.

Following is one method for massaging the male G-spot. Consider using a finger cot (a latex cover for a finger) or a latex glove. Whether you choose a bare or gloved finger, use lots of lubrication! Or use a lubricated sex toy with a flared base (so it doesn't get lost inside the rectum). Insert your finger or anal sex toy slowly and gently into your partner's anus. Ask him to bear down slightly (as though pushing out a bowel movement) to ease the entry of your finger or the toy. Let him guide you verbally on when and how to continue. Let the sphincter muscle (about one inch up the rectum) relax before you insert more.

- If you're using a finger, once you are inside past your second knuckle, make a gentle "come here" signal toward his belly button. You should feel a round sphere, which is the prostate.
- Keep making a slow, gentle, curving in-and-out motion. Be careful not to use the edge of your nail—stick to the pads of your fingers, which are softer. When your partner has indicated he has had enough, slowly withdraw your finger or the toy as you inserted it. If he has had an orgasm, the pubococcygeal muscle will have tightened, so be aware that you may have some tightness upon pulling out.

Entering Vaginas

Have you ever seen a movie sex scene in which a man climbs on top of a woman and pumps like crazy for what seems like hours while she is having orgasm after orgasm, thrashing about and moaning out her lover's name? Yeah, me too. But it's not reality.

Scenarios like that can be downright intimidating, and they can create pressure on men to live up to unreasonable sexual standards, which may result in performance anxiety, an inability to achieve or maintain an erection, or delayed or inhibited ejaculation.

The bottom line is that most women do not orgasm from vaginal penetration alone; most need clitoral stimulation either on its own or in conjunction with penetration.

Safer Penetration

Unprotected penile-vaginal penetration can put you at risk for any number of sexually transmitted infections, including HIV, herpes, genital warts, gonorrhea, syphilis, hepatitis B, parasites (such as crabs), and chlamydia. Correctly and consistently using a latex or polyurethane condom can greatly reduce your risk of infection and unintended pregnancy.

Although no condom guarantees 100 percent protection against failure, most condom failures result mainly from human error, including improper storage or use. Here are some tips to help you get the most comfort and security out of your condom:

- **Store your condoms in a cool, dark place. Exposure to sunlight, heat, or humidity can break down latex, causing it to tear more easily.**
- **Always check the date on the box or on the back of an individual condom package. Some dates are marked "MFG," which indicates the manufacturing date. These condoms are good up to four years from the MFG date. Others are marked "EXP," which indicates the date after which the condom should not be used. If you are unsure how old the condom is, throw it away and use a new one.**
- **Lambskin condoms or natural condoms are not effective in the prevention of disease. For the best protection, be sure to use only latex condoms.**

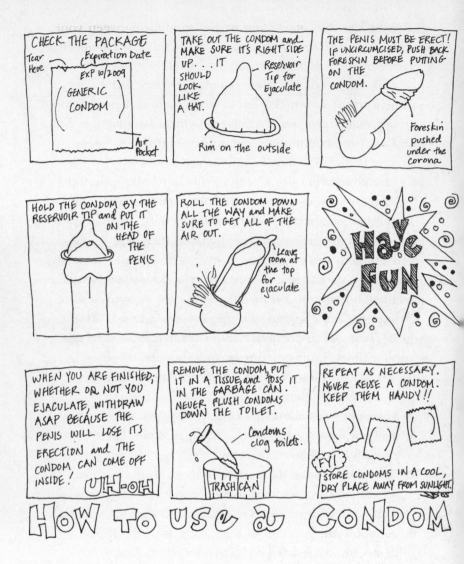

- Be careful when opening a condom package that you do not tear or nick the latex with your teeth, nails, or rings. Do not unroll the condom before putting it on; it can weaken the latex and make it difficult to use.

- Hold the receptacle end of the condom between your thumb and forefinger against the head of the penis. If the penis is uncircumcised, pull back the foreskin first. Make sure to leave space at the tip so the semen will not leak out the side of the condom. *Squeeze out any excess air to prevent the condom from bursting.*
- Roll the condom over the entire length of the penis.
- Use plenty of water-based lubricant during intercourse. Putting a drop of lubricant inside the tip of the condom can increase both sensation and safety. Oil-based lubricants, like petroleum jelly, baby oil, and lotion, will diminish the strength of latex 70 percent in less than thirty seconds!
- After you are finished, pull out while the penis is still hard, holding on to the base of the condom to prevent it from falling off. Roll it gently toward the tip of the penis to remove. If you have ejaculated, be careful not to spill any of it on your partner's genitals.
- Do not flush condoms down the toilet because they can clog plumbing. Wrap in a tissue and throw away. Remember, condoms cannot be reused.

What did you learn in this chapter?

_____

_____

What did you read that surprised you?

_____

_____

What would you like to learn more about?

_____

_____

Something I learned about penises and testicles from reading this chapter is:

_____

_____

FOR THOSE WITH PENISES

Some love their penises, some don't give it much thought, and others have penis complaints. The following worksheet will help you figure out how you feel about your penis.

What name or nickname do you use for your
penis? _____

What do you call it when you are with an intimate
partner? _____

What do you call it when you are at the doctor's office? _____

What do you prefer to have it called? _____

The following words describe my penis (check all that apply):

Attractive	❑	Uncircumcised	❑
Normal	❑	Weird	❑
Ugly	❑	Strong	❑
A good size	❑	Skinny	❑
Smaller than I would like	❑	Hefty	❑
Bigger than I would like	❑	Sexy	❑
Curvy	❑	Hot	❑
Circumcised	❑	Other:	_____

The best thing about my penis is:

_____

_____

If there was one thing I could change about my penis, it would be:

_____

_____

I have tasted my semen   ❏

My semen tastes like:_____

My semen smells like: _____

My semen looks like:_____

I have never tasted my semen   ❏

Why not?

_____

Partners have given me the following compliments about my penis:

_____

_____

My penis enjoys the following activities:

❏   Oral sex (fellatio)

Describe what you like:

_____

_____

❑   Penetrating a vagina
Describe what you like:
_____
_____

❑   Penetrating an anus
Describe what you like:
_____
_____

❑   Hand job
Describe what you like:
_____
_____

❑   Penetrating _____ (insert object, person, thing)
Describe what you like:
_____
_____

My penis also enjoys:
_____
_____

Chapter 8

SELF-SEXPLORATION

*Masturbation and
Other Self-Pleasuring*

✳ ✳ ✳

*I masturbate, and I agree with whoever it was that gave the
arguments for it: it's free, it's always available, you can't get
anybody pregnant, you can't get any diseases—and you meet a
better class of people.*
—Quote from a seventy-two-year-old man in the book
*Older and Wiser: Wit, Wisdom, and Spirited Advice
from the Older Generation*

What do Kellogg's cornflakes and graham crackers have
in common? These tasty products were originally invented in the 1800s as bland foods to lessen people's sex drive
and reduce masturbation, which was seen as deviant and linked
to physical and psychological illness. Kellogg and Graham
both contributed to a long legacy of misinformation, guilt, and
pleasure-phobic attitudes about masturbation (also called *auto-
eroticism* or *sex for one*). In 1966, Masters & Johnson "revealed"
that masturbation cuts across all boundaries of sex, age, race,

and social class, and in 1972, the American Medical Association declared masturbation a "normal" sexual activity. So it's official: There is nothing unnatural about masturbation!

Masturbation is the best way to learn about your body and its sexual responsiveness—what feels good, where it feels good, and how it feels good. There is no performance anxiety or expectations because it is just you. You can take your time or be as speedy as you care to be. You can experiment with all kinds of things that you may not feel comfortable doing right away (or ever) with someone else, and you can use that information for yourself or share it with a partner.

Self-pleasuring allows people to focus on their own needs—even when they are in a sexual relationship. Masturbation provides a sexual outlet for couples when they are apart, when one partner is ill, when one partner is not interested in sex, or when either partner cannot get enough stimulation through sexual intercourse to reach orgasm.

First Self-Sexplorations

Doting parents often coo to their toddler, "Point to your nose," "Point to your tummy," but it is the rare parent who will add, "Show Mommy where your penis is," and clap gleefully when the child touches it. Babies like to touch their genitals for the same reason they like to be bathed and cuddled. It feels nice, plain and simple. Your toddler probably is not fantasizing about a crazy sex weekend. He is probably thinking, "I'm hungry, I'm thirsty, I'm tired, Ooo this blankie is cozy, I'm sad, I'm happy, Where's Mommy, Hey, here's my penis." Many children learn that the genitals are private or dirty and definitely not to be played with. Nevertheless, plenty of people discover the wonders of genital self-exploration.

When little girls are toilet trained, they are taught to wipe themselves with a piece of toilet paper. Unlike boys, girls have nothing hanging out that they can readily see. So they rarely see or touch the skin of their genitals. Girls may "accidentally" discover the pleasure derived from touching their genitals while bathing or standing under the shower nozzle, for example. They may discover that rubbing against stuffed animals, blankets, or pieces of furniture feels good.

For me it started in second grade. I was the best rope climber in my gym class. I'd always be the first one to volunteer to climb. I would wrap my legs around the rope and pull on my arms to help me get all the way to the top. It always felt so good on the way up. Usually, by the time I got to the top it felt super-good and sometimes super-duper good. For some reason unbeknownst to me, my arms and legs always felt a bit jellylike on the way down.

When I mentioned to my younger brother my amazing discovery of the power of rope climbing, he just couldn't relate. "I don't feel anything," he said. "Maybe you're not doing it right," I said. Nope. He just never got it. Now I know why. I was masturbating on the ropes and having orgasms as I got to the top.

For my brother, however, squeezing his legs together, having tension in his arms, and rubbing his crotch against the rope was not stimulating. I didn't share my technique with anyone else; somehow I knew that what I was doing was something I shouldn't share with others. I felt it was wrong, but I didn't really know why. But it didn't stop me. And I was not alone in this pursuit.

Nia, thirty-eight, discovered when she was eight or nine years old that if she climbed on the back of the couch and moved back and forth, it would feel really good. As she describes it, *"I would pretend I was on a horse and told my mother I was playing cowgirl. Ride 'em, horsie!"*

Kelsey, thirty, would press against the edge of the closet door in her bedroom: *"It started when I was about eight years old. I would grip both door handles and move up and down. When I started having sex with a man, I had trouble having orgasms until we tried a position that simulated the one on the door. He stood up and I wrapped my arms and legs around him and moved up and down. I was relieved that all those years of door humping hadn't destroyed my ability to have an orgasm with a guy. Sometimes I still hump the door when I want to masturbate."*

Shannon, thirty-two, who grew up with four brothers, explains that in her family, it was expected that guys masturbate: *"My parents used to joke around with my older brothers when they were spending a lot of time in the bathroom. They'd knock on the door and say, 'You must be whacking off in there, are you finished yet?' No one ever said anything about me masturbating. I got the message that it was okay for guys to do it, but not for girls."*

Some women actually learn how to masturbate from a partner—by practicing the way in which they were manually stimulated. Jessica, forty-five, was sexually naive when she was younger and learned about masturbation techniques from her first boyfriend: *"I had only masturbated by rubbing against a pillow while lying on my stomach. The first time that David and I went to 'third base,' he put a finger inside my vagina and wiggled it around. I was amazed at how good it felt. It had never occurred to me to do something like that! David didn't last, but his technique certainly did."*

The first time Hannah, thirty-nine, masturbated was in college: *"I was taking a women's-studies course and we read* Our Bodies, Ourselves *for class. After reading about all of those enlightened women, I was determined to have an orgasm by myself. I waited until my roommate was out, got out my copy of the book, and tried different techniques until one worked. I felt totally empowered."*

Male genitalia, however, are external—easily seen and accessible and impossible to ignore. When boys are toilet trained, they are encouraged to hold their penis to better aim into the toilet.

When they touch their penises, boys may "learn" how pleasurable self-touch can be. This may be one reason why they are more comfortable self-sexploring.

Gordon, twenty-one, describes his first foray into masturbation: *"Well, when I was probably around the age of twelve, I was super curious about sex. So I would sneak into the school library and steal the books on sex and development (I didn't want to take them out so that there was a paper trail!), but that wasn't enough. At a used-book sale at the public library, I discovered just what I needed—an adult's guide to sexuality! I found the chapter on masturbation and tried it out. The dryness led to chafing, and being undeveloped, I simply bled upon climax, with no ejaculation. But from that point on, I was determined to develop this newfound skill and please myself. With the help of Web sites and books, I was able to learn various techniques and master masturbation."*

Sam recalls, *"When I was thirteen, I broke my arm and had to learn how to use my other hand to jerk off. My mom was concerned about me learning to write and brush my teeth with my left hand, but I was in a crisis because I was a right-handed masturbator!"*

What are your memories about self-sexploration? Did your experience include confusion and misinformation (see "Masturbation Myths and Facts," page 156)? Shame or embarrassment? Excitement and satisfaction? Write about your experiences below.

_____

_____

_____

Would you consider the impact of your experience to be positive, negative, or unknown? Why?

_____

_____

How does your experience with masturbation impact on your adult sexuality?

MasturMind

*H*ow you feel about masturbation is for you to decide. As far as your body is concerned, no part of you is inherently dirty, evil, or untouchable. The skin on your penis or vulva has the identical structure as the skin on your neck or arms; it's just in a different anatomical location. Yet many people consider their genitals "dirty" and "shameful." Your sex organs don't know and don't care who or what is the source of their stimulation. Most young men experience spontaneous erections when they are not consciously thinking sexual thoughts or doing anything to stimulate themselves. The male body does not know or care whether its semen ends up in a vagina or a throat or an anal cavity or in a towel. The female body doesn't care whether its own hand, the hand of another, or a vibrator stimulates it. Basically, your body doesn't judge its reaction . . . that happens in your mind.

If your parent or caregiver slapped your hand or scolded you when you touched yourself, you may think masturbation is "dirty" and are ashamed of masturbating. For some people, religious teachings may be a source of conflict about masturbation. Maybe you learned in religious school that masturbation was "sinful." Maybe you heard myths about masturbation, such as you could go blind or your penis would fall off or you wouldn't be a virgin anymore if you masturbated (see box on page 156). It's no wonder that masturbation can be such an uncomfortable topic to discuss.

Yet plenty of people happily view masturbation as "self-loving" and enjoy the pleasure they achieve. Melissa, twenty-four, when playing with the "boys" (as she refers to her vibrators), will often encourage herself with a "Yes, that's the spot, you've got it now!"

Others have tried masturbating, don't feel bad about it, but don't much like it. That's fine, too. Yet statistics show that no matter how they feel about it, most men and women choose to masturbate. As a matter of fact, it is estimated that up to 80 percent of women and 94 percent of men between the ages of eighteen and forty-nine years old masturbate.

Some do it and feel guilty. Some feel no guilt but are definitely "underground" about masturbating and wouldn't admit to doing it no matter who asked them. Others revel in their masturbation, happily telling others about their techniques. Some will tell a select few people that they masturbate but may feel uncomfortable telling an intimate partner. Basically, we display a variety of actions and feelings around masturbation. They are all normal.

Sarina, thirty-three, describes how her feelings about masturbation stemmed from reading *The Story of O*: *"I read and reread O and hid it under my pillow. In one section of the book, O's master asks her to masturbate. She tries to touch herself. But even though she will do anything else he asks, she just cannot bring herself to do that. So my lesson was that sexually desirable adult women would not consider degrading themselves in this way, even though they would be naked and penetrated and bound and beaten at the drop of a hat. That left me very confused."*

"As far as self-pleasuring, I'd always viewed it as a 'lonely' thing to do, that doing it was sad, so I didn't. One of my boyfriends convinced me to do it in front of him, and it opened up a whole new world!" Margarita, forty-two.

Who masturbates? Single people masturbate, people in casual relationships masturbate, people in committed relationships masturbate, and those who are divorced or widowed masturbate. Children, teenagers, adults, and the elderly masturbate. People who identify as straight, gay, lesbian, bisexual, asexual, or trans-gender masturbate. People of different religious and cultural backgrounds masturbate. Masturbation is the great equalizer!

Masturbation can provide sexual satisfaction for people who are without a partner for whatever reason. There are all kinds of people who are not with partners—some out of choice, some because they're waiting for the right person, some because of religious beliefs, and some because they are in nursing homes or physically incapacitated.

Yelena, twenty-eight, says, *"Judy Blume definitely helped shape my views on masturbation. Reading* Deenie *as an eleven-year-old girl with scoliosis and learning that Deenie, a fourteen-year-old girl with scoliosis, touched her special place at night and that this was okay, vali-dated something that was definitely murky in my mind."*

For Jose, as a fifteen-year-old who was dating a boy who lived on the other side of town, the problem of neither of them hav-ing a driver's license led them to masturbation within a relation-ship: *"During our week- or multiple week-long separations, when we spoke on the phone for hours a night, it simply evolved. In our late night phone conversations, as we each lay in our rooms miles apart, we would pleasure ourselves and share the experience."*

Ingrid, twenty-five, doesn't feel comfortable masturbating but will do so during phone sex with her boyfriend: *"I'm doing it, but I'm sharing it, so it doesn't feel so selfish to me. And I know it's getting him off, too."*

How Often Do People Masturbate?

There is no "normal" frequency of masturbation. Some do it every day, even several times a day. Some do it infrequently or use it to relieve stress. Some people masturbate at certain times of the month when their sex drive is stronger. It varies, and it's all okay. As long as masturbation doesn't interfere with your daily activities and your interpersonal interactions, do it as often as you want. If you do little else besides masturbate or you consistently avoid going out with friends so that you can stay home and masturbate, then you may want to talk to a counselor or a medical provider about what you're doing.

"It really takes just a photo or a glimpse of a vagina to make me hard and want to jack off. Between erotic photos, videos, and putting my face between my partner's legs, I figure I masturbate between two and three times per day while looking at vaginas, as close up as I can. That's at least one thousand times per year, for every year since I was twelve, and I am in my late forties now." Larry, forty-eight.

Where Are People's Mastur-Places?

𝒪ne of the best things about masturbation is that it's a portable activity. It can be private or public. People masturbate on the subway, on a plane, in a car, in their office at work, in the bathroom, and—most typically—in their bedroom. Of course, there are decency laws, so public genital displays can be illegal. Hey, not everyone is into exhibitionism.

For Katherine, forty-one, privacy is key, and a relaxing bath is the ultimate setting: *"I light candles, put on Barry White, and relax. I like to run my hands over my body and 'tease myself' before I get to work. Setting the mood makes it much more pleasurable for me."*

Sometimes you get the urge to masturbate when the time or place just isn't convenient. What can you do? Maybe a quick masturbation in a bathroom is the answer. Consistently masturbating quickly, however, can have lasting consequences. Sanjay, twenty, was concerned about premature ejaculation, even though he had never had penetrative intercourse. During our discussion, he described how most of his experiences involved locking himself in the bathroom at home and working as quickly as he could to come so that he wouldn't get caught. So basically he trained himself to come fast. He was worried that when he had partner sex he would come too quickly. I encouraged him to practice using the "squeeze technique" to delay ejaculation. He said, "Now those are the types of practice sessions that I can really get into!" The squeeze technique is one method used to delay ejaculation, particularly for those who tend to ejaculate more quickly than they would like. When you are close to orgasm, take the penis between your thumb and first two fingers, press your thumb against the prepuce (the little muscle under the head where the foreskin is or was attached) and squeeze, gently but firmly, for three or four seconds.

For those who do not live alone, finding masturbation time at home can be challenging. Brian, twenty-eight, majored in acting in college: *"I was literally gone from my room from eight o'clock in the morning until midnight. I would crawl into bed only to be awakened at four a.m. by my roommate jerking off. I was so pissed. I mean, I was gone for sixteen hours a day and he couldn't find another time to jerk off?"*

Well, it's certainly possible that Brian's roommate got off on getting off when there was someone else around, but unless you have someone's consent to do so, you should never force your masturbation on anyone else. If, on the other hand, you want to have some privacy for your solo adventures, you may have to get creative. Here are some tips for those with roommates or other live-in partners:

- Post your schedules or have a calendar to keep track of everyone's plans. This allows roommates to see when they'll have the place to themselves. Keep in mind that plans can change and someone can return unexpectedly.
- Tell each other how long you'll be gone when you're going out. A simple "I'm going out for a long, leisurely dinner" or "I'm going to pick up the mail downstairs" will help let you know how much alone time you have.

- Some people masturbate with their clothes on. Many women enjoy masturbating in jeans because of the heavy stitching and hard zipper in the genital area. Some like to use a maxipad under their clothes when doing this so that their underwear doesn't get wet.
- Make knocking a regular part of entering your room.

Master or Mistress of Your Domain

*B*oth men and women can use masturbation to explore what turns them on by experimenting with various body parts, different ways of touching, inserting or using different objects, differing speeds and pressures, and engaging in fantasies. There is no right or wrong way to do it, and the way you do it can change over time, or you can stick with the tried-and-true methods you've been using since childhood. I won't be going over all the possibilities—otherwise this book would be very long—but we'll talk about some basic techniques and a few variations. Although masturbation methods differ for men and women, there are common elements for both. Use the worksheet for women (page 158) or the worksheet for men (page 166) to aid you in your self-sexploration. It's a tool to help you figure out what you like, how you like it, where and when you like it, and in what ways you want to experiment in the future. You can keep the information to yourself or share it with a partner so that he or she knows what you like to do (and maybe can do those things with you or to you). "Mastur" the possibilities!

I'm in the Mood for *Self*-Love . . .

*S*etting the mood for masturbation can be a key element for your ultimate enjoyment. How about some candlelight and jazz? Perhaps you like daylight and indie rock. Maybe you want to watch yourself in the mirror or stand in front of the television. Sometimes a long, hot shower is just what the doctor ordered. Whatever, whenever, try to create an environment that provides comfort and allows you freedom from the stress of your life.

Not every masturbation session needs to end in orgasm or ejaculation; that should not always be the ultimate goal. Sometimes it's relaxing just to touch yourself or play with your genitals. There is no pressure to "perform," especially when you are alone.

Mastur-Male

*N*o matter what you call it—jerking, jacking, whacking or getting off, spilling the sperm, shooting your wad, spanking the monkey, diddling, slapping the salami, or yanking the chain—it's all male masturbation. And male masturbation techniques are as varied as the men who perform them.

The most common position for men is lying on their back and rubbing their penis with a hand (or hands). Jackin' World (www.jackinworld.com), a great Web site with hundreds of masturbation techniques for men, offers the following four basic ways to grip your penis during masturbation.

The Fist
In this technique, you wrap your fingers around the shaft of the penis as if you're holding a baseball bat and rub up and down. This technique provides the most contact between your hand and the penis. More surface area covered equals more pleasure. This technique is particularly recommended for those with larger penises, because holding on with your whole hand leaves less room for moving your hand up and down.

The Five-Finger

In this technique, your hand and arm form an angle with your penis, with four fingers on top of the shaft at a diagonal and your thumb below. This allows you to get more control over the hand-to-penis contact, and it lets you move your hand along the entire length of the shaft, even if your penis isn't very large.

The Three-Finger

This one is good if you have a smaller penis. Simply hold the penis as you would a pen or pencil. This grip allows maximum control and maximum distance of motion (from the base of the penis all the way to the head), but the hand-to-penis contact is less than with the other grips.

The Backhand

This one, kind of a backward version of "the fist," is a little funny, but it feels very good. This time, grab your penis from the left side rather than the right (or vice versa if you're left-handed). To do this, rotate your wrist so that your thumb is pointing down; you may have to pull your penis slightly to the side. It's a little awkward at first, but it's an excellent grip to use when you want to try something other than "the fist" for a few minutes.

One of the most important components of masturbation is lubrication. You can never have enough lube! Lube up your hands and your penis with your own saliva; water-based lubricants such as ID, Astroglide, or KY; silicone-based lubricants such as Eros; or petroleum-based products such as vaseline. You can also try yummy food products such as yogurt, jelly, chocolate sauce, and mashed bananas.

Men can use their hands to manually stimulate the shaft and/or head of the penis in a variety of ways. They can enclose the head of the penis with one hand while stroking up and down with the other. They can slap the penis back and forth steadily between their hands (hence the term *beating off*), rub against an object or another body part, or insert their penis into an object. They can also touch, rub, or hold their testicles or perineum (the area between the testicles and the anus— sometimes called the male G-spot) and stroke or insert a finger or other object into their anus (just make sure it has a wide base and can't get lost inside!). The prostate gland can be stimulated through the anus (see page 133 for more information about anal stimulation) and lead to orgasm.

Mastur-Female

𝒪t is more common for women to be preorgasmic (that is, to have never experienced an orgasm) than it is for men. A good thing to buy, if you are a preorgasmic woman, is a plug-in vibrator such as a Hitachi Magic Wand. This, possibly together with one of Betty Dodson's books or videotapes (*Sex for One* or *Self Loving*) or Carol Queen's videotape on vibrators (*Carol Queen's Great Vibrations*), should set you on the right track. The key is just to have fun without being too goal oriented.

Women can use their fingers and hands to stimulate their vulva (mons pubis, clitoris, vaginal lips, and vagina), perineum, and anus. Women use vibrators and/or dildos, running water, and the act of rubbing their vulvas against a pillow, a chair, or the floor and may insert objects into the vagina to masturbate.

Some women start out slowly, lightly touching their inner and outer lips, clitoris, and vagina and languishing for an hour or more. Others get right to work, going straight for the orgasm.

Starting on the outside, you may use your fingers, the palm of your hand, or a feather and play around with the sensations, moving faster or slower, harder or softer, stroking or squeezing for variety. If touching the clitoris directly is too intense for you, rub on either side or use your middle and index finger in a V position on either side. Try rubbing with an open hand over the entire vulva area, or lie on your stomach and rub against some object such as a pillow. Another method of clitoral stimulation is using a shower massage so that a pulsating (or steady) stream of water washes over the vulva and clitoris. Be sure to keep the water temperature low enough so that you don't burn yourself. Of course, the ever popular vibrator provides one hell of a dependable orgasm for many women (see page 226 for more about sex toys).

Some women will keep their playing only on the outside of their genitals. Others may venture into the vaginal canal, usually in conjunction with clitoral stimulation. You can insert one finger or two or three or even your entire hand. Moving fingers around inside the vaginal canal can feel great. Inserting objects such as vibrators, dildos, or the handle of some tool can give a different sensation. Some women like to wiggle the objects inside, some like to move the objects in and out, and some use these objects to stimulate their G-spot (see page 100 for how to find the G-spot).

Here are a few safety tips to keep in mind when using objects for masturbation:

- **Clean your toys. Objects inserted vaginally/anally need to be washed with hot soapy water after each use. Unplug and/or take the batteries out of any electrical toys before washing them.**
- **Toys and objects for insertion must be sturdy and not easily broken; long enough to have a "handle," or a flared base, so that they can't get stuck inside; and**

MASTURBATION MYTHS AND FACTS

MYTH: I will go blind or insane.

FACT: These ideas gained popularity in America in the 1800s. It was believed, in error, that masturbation depleted a person's energy so severely that it weakened his or her nervous system, which affected a person's health in general. Masturbation was believed to lead to health problems, like loss of vision and sanity. Today we know that engaging in masturbation contributes positively to our well-being and good health.

MYTH: I will grow hair on my palms.

FACT: So the hair from your head moves to your palms?! Seriously, a person is likely to masturbate at about the time hair starts growing on various parts of the body that didn't have hair before. This is due to hormones, not touching your genitals.

MYTH: I will get acne.

FACT: Masturbation does *not* cause pimples. But some people might think so because the hormones that cause the development of sexual urges are also the hormones likely to cause skin problems. This is a case of faulty cause-and-effect reasoning.

MYTH: My penis will turn green and fall off.

FACT: Frequent and vigorous masturbation can produce skin abrasions. That will make your penis redden—but it won't fall off. Using KY jelly, Aqua Lube, saliva, or even soap and water can help you avoid abrasion.

MYTH: I won't be a virgin anymore.

FACT: Everyone has a different view of what it means to be a virgin. But most people agree that loss of virginity involves having sex with a partner. Any act of self-penetration could stretch your hymen, but then so can riding a horse, using a tampon, or doing gymnastics—and most equestrians would agree they are in no way having sex with their horses!

MYTH: My sperm will be "wasted."

FACT: The testicles produce semen at the rate of thousands of sperm a second. Reservoirs near the prostate gland are being refilled continuously.

Each ejaculation partially empties the chambers, but more sperm will arrive to refill them. If they are not emptied by masturbation or intercourse, they will be voided automatically during sleep in the form of nocturnal emissions or naturally reabsorbed by the body.

MYTH: Masturbating too frequently will lower one's sperm count.

FACT: Men cannot "run out" of sperm (any more than you can "run out" of other fluids your body produces, like saliva), so they can masturbate as often as they like. The worst thing that can happen is your penis might get a little sore. (Rub any part of your body that much and the same thing will happen!)

MYTH: If I masturbate, I won't be able to orgasm with a partner.

FACT: Actually, masturbating can greatly improve your ability to have an orgasm with a partner. Since we are all different, there is no way that someone can know what you like unless you let him or her know. Learning what you like will enable you to help your partner help you to have better partner sex.

MYTH: If my partner masturbates, it is because he or she is not satisfied with our sex life.

FACT: Masturbation has nothing to do with partner satisfaction. Most people feel that masturbation is pleasurable in a different way from partner sex. You might like cake and steak, but you wouldn't want to give up one for the other because both fill different needs. In fact, some people find they actually masturbate more when they are engaged in a fulfilling sex life with a partner because their sexual senses are heightened.

closed at the end, because the internal suction created by an open bottle, for example, can cause damage to internal organs.

• Be careful to maintain a balanced water temperature when using a stream of water—water that is too hot or too cold (or ice) can be damaging to genital tissue.

THE BENEFITS OF MASTURBATION

- You can indulge in harmless, pleasurable sexual fantasies and explore what turns you on without tending to a partner's needs.
- You can reduce stress and sexual tension. After masturbation, many people experience a pleasant, tranquil feeling due to the release of certain chemicals into the bloodstream (which is why some paraplegics who cannot feel their sex organs can nonetheless enjoy sex). These chemicals induce a quiet and relaxed state after sex, which some people interpret as sleepiness.
- It can help you become more comfortable with your own sexuality, learning what you like and how you like to be touched.
- It can be enjoyable when shared with a partner.
- You won't get pregnant or contract a sexually transmitted infection by masturbating. It's the safest form of safer sex!
- It can relieve some physical discomfort (such as menstrual cramps).
- It can be energizing.
- Once you know how to make yourself orgasm, it can be a lot easier to teach a partner how to make you come.
- It's economical, free, time-saving, and almost always available!

MASTURBATION WORKSHEET FOR WOMEN

Use this worksheet for self-sexploration about masturbation. You may want to keep it for yourself, or you may choose to share it with a partner (you can exchange worksheets if you want) to let him or her know your likes and dislikes and what you'd like to try in the future.

MY MASTURBATION HISTORY
Write a few lines about the role that masturbation has or has not played in your life.

Age when I first masturbated: _____

Messages I received about masturbation from:
Parents _____
Religious leaders _____
School _____
Community _____
Friends_____
Partners _____
Movies/books/TV _____
Other _____

What are some myths that you heard about masturbation growing up?
1) _____
2) _____
3) _____

What is one positive masturbation memory?
_____
_____

What is one not so positive masturbation memory?
_____
_____

Slang terms I use for masturbation:

_____

_____

Write a few lines about the role that masturbation has or has not played in your life. Include the age at which you first masturbated, if at all, any reaction from grown-ups that you remember, what you learned about it from books, movies, or others in your life, myths you may have heard, and anything else you would like to add.

_____

_____

_____

GETTING TO KNOW ME
Do you know what your vulva looks like? The best way to see it is to hold a mirror in one hand, lie down on a bed or other comfortable place, and place the mirror facing your vulva. Use your other hand to spread your outer vulva lips so that you can see the inner lips and the outside nub of the clitoris (see "Vulvar Self-Exam" in chapter 6). Draw a picture of your vulva here:

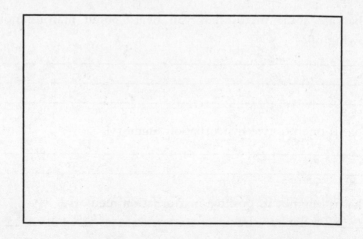

Use the picture on the previous page as your personal vulva pleasure map. Label the following on your picture:

"★" for the parts that feel good when you touch them.

"☺" for the parts that are ticklish.

"x" for the parts that feel uncomfortable when touched.

You can do the same thing for your vagina and for other parts of your body like your feet, neck, breasts, and so forth.

FEELINGS ABOUT MASTURBATION

It may be helpful for you to assess your current feelings about masturbating in order to help you understand your comfort level about solo sex.

	Agree	Disagree	Don't Know
Masturbation is normal	❏	❏	❏
I feel comfortable masturbating	❏	❏	❏
I would never tell anyone that I masturbate	❏	❏	❏
Masturbation isn't sex	❏	❏	❏
People in relationships shouldn't have to do it	❏	❏	❏
Masturbation is beneficial to your health	❏	❏	❏
Vibrators are for people with sexual problems	❏	❏	❏
Men need to masturbate more than women	❏	❏	❏
It's okay to masturbate in front of your partner	❏	❏	❏
I feel guilty when I masturbate	❏	❏	❏
I wouldn't masturbate if I had a sexual partner	❏	❏	❏

Orgasms with masturbation
   aren't as good   ❏   ❏   ❏

REASONS FOR MASTURBATING
Here are some reasons why women masturbate. Check off the
ones that apply to you.

I'm not having sex with anyone else right now   ❏
I prefer to have sex with myself   ❏
I use it as a method of safer sex   ❏
I use it as a method of birth control   ❏
Sex with a partner never brings me to orgasm   ❏
I like the orgasms that I have when I masturbate ❏
It relieves tension   ❏
No one pleases me better than me   ❏
It's easier to come when I do it myself   ❏
I can do it anytime, anywhere   ❏
My partner doesn't like to use sex toys   ❏
I don't want my partner to
   know that I like sex toys   ❏
Other:
_____

_____

REASONS FOR NOT MASTURBATING
Here are some reasons why women don't masturbate. Check
off the ones that apply to you.

Uncomfortable touching myself   ❏
Religious beliefs   ❏
Don't know how to do it   ❏
Feel guilty   ❏
Am ashamed   ❏
Don't want to do it   ❏
Tried it and didn't like it   ❏

Tried it and couldn't orgasm ❑
No privacy ❑
Don't think it's necessary ❑
Don't think it's important to do ❑
Don't care about it ❑
Rather do it with a partner ❑
Other:

_____

_____

PLACES I MASTURBATE

	Do it	Want to try	Maybe	No way
In my bed	❑	❑	❑	❑
In the bathroom/ shower/bathtub	❑	❑	❑	❑
In the car	❑	❑	❑	❑
At work	❑	❑	❑	❑
At the movies	❑	❑	❑	❑
In a hotel room	❑	❑	❑	❑

Other:

_____

_____

MASTURBATION TECHNIQUES (SEE PAGES 154–157 FOR MORE SPECIFIC DESCRIPTIONS OF THESE TECHNIQUES)

	Do it	Want to try	Maybe	No way
One hand outside	❑	❑	❑	❑
Two hands outside	❑	❑	❑	❑
One hand outside/ finger inside	❑	❑	❑	❑

	Do it	Want to try	Maybe	No way
V-stroke on clitoris	❑	❑	❑	❑
Using a vibrator without inserting it	❑	❑	❑	❑
Vibrator inserted	❑	❑	❑	❑
Dildo or other object inserted	❑	❑	❑	❑
Under running water	❑	❑	❑	❑
Rubbing on a towel, pillow, stuffed toy, etc.	❑	❑	❑	❑
Rubbing against edge of a chair, a door, etc	❑	❑	❑	❑
Sitting on the washing machine or dryer	❑	❑	❑	❑
Squeezing my legs together	❑	❑	❑	❑

Other:

_____

_____

MY PREFERRED MASTURBATION ENVIRONMENT
Check off all that apply.

Dark room ❑
Music playing ❑   Type of music:_____
No one home ❑
Other people around ❑

Bedtime ❏
Morning ❏
Fifteen-minute work break ❏
Watching erotica/porn ❏ Favorite videos:_____
Reading erotica/porn ❏ Favorite erotica/porn:
Fantasizing ❏ _____
Candles burning ❏
Shades or curtains closed ❏
Shades or curtains open ❏
Quiet ❏
Other:

_____

_____

SOUNDS I MAKE

	Always	Sometimes	Never	Maybe someday
No sound at all	❏	❏	❏	❏
Moan softly	❏	❏	❏	❏
Moan loudly	❏	❏	❏	❏
Have escalating moans	❏	❏	❏	❏
Breathe heavily	❏	❏	❏	❏
Pant	❏	❏	❏	❏
Scream	❏	❏	❏	❏
Cry	❏	❏	❏	❏
Laugh	❏	❏	❏	❏
Sing	❏	❏	❏	❏
Hold my breath	❏	❏	❏	❏
Call someone's name	❏	❏	❏	❏

Other:

_____

_____

MY MASTURBATION FANTASY

_____

_____

_____

_____

What did you learn from doing this worksheet?

_____

_____

MASTURBATION WORKSHEET FOR MEN

Use this worksheet for self-exploration about masturbation. You may want to keep it for yourself, or you may choose to share it with a partner (you can exchange worksheets if you want) to let him or her know your likes and dislikes and what you'd like to try in the future.

MY MASTURBATION HISTORY
Write a few lines about the role that masturbation has or has not played in your life.

Age when I first masturbated: _____

Messages I received about masturbation from:
Parents _____
Religious leaders _____
School _____
Community_____
Friends_____
Partners _____
Movies/books/TV _____
Other _____

What are some myths that you heard about masturbation growing up?

1) _____

2) _____

3) _____

What is one positive masturbation memory?

_____

_____

What is one not so positive masturbation memory?

_____

_____

Slang terms I use for masturbation:

_____

_____

_____

GETTING TO KNOW ME

It's time to take a good look at your penis and testicles in both its flaccid (non-erect) and erect states. Stand in front of the mirror and draw what you see. A lot of men have morning erections, so keep a pencil handy in the a.m. (see "Penis Picture Show" on page 121). Draw a picture of your penis and testicles on the next page (don't forget the foreskin, if you have it).

Flaccid	Erect

Use the picture above as your personal penile pleasure map. Label the following on your picture:

"★" for the parts that feel good when you touch them.
"☺" for the parts that are ticklish.
"x" for the parts that feel uncomfortable when touched.

You can do the same thing for your testicles and for other parts of your body like your feet, neck, chest, and so forth.

FEELINGS ABOUT MASTURBATION
It may be helpful for you to assess your current feelings about masturbating in order to help you understand your comfort level about solo sex.

	Agree	Disagree	Don't know
Masturbation is normal	❑	❑	❑
I feel comfortable masturbating	❑	❑	❑

	Agree	Disagree	Don't know
I would never tell anyone that I masturbate	❑	❑	❑
Masturbation isn't sex	❑	❑	❑
People in relationships shouldn't have to do it	❑	❑	❑
Masturbation is beneficial to your health	❑	❑	❑
Sex toys are for those with sexual problems	❑	❑	❑
Men need to masturbate more than women	❑	❑	❑
It's okay to masturbate in front of your partner	❑	❑	❑
I feel guilty when I masturbate	❑	❑	❑
I wouldn't masturbate if I had a sexual partner	❑	❑	❑
Orgasms with masturbation aren't as good	❑	❑	❑

REASONS FOR MASTURBATING

Here are some reasons why men masturbate. Check off the ones that apply to you.

I'm not having sex with anyone else right now	❑
I prefer to have sex with myself	❑
I use it as a method of safer sex	❑
I use it as a method of birth control	❑
Sex with a partner never brings me to orgasm	❑
I like the orgasms that I have when I masturbate	❑
It relieves tension	❑

No one pleases me better than me ❑
It's easier to come when I do it myself ❑
I can do it anytime, anywhere ❑
My partner doesn't get me off ❑
I don't want my partner to know that I like kinky ❑
Other:

_____

_____

REASONS FOR NOT MASTURBATING
Here are some reasons why men don't masturbate. Check off the ones that apply to you.

Uncomfortable touching myself ❑
Religious beliefs ❑
Don't know how to do it ❑
Feel guilty ❑
Am ashamed ❑
Don't want to do it ❑
Tried it and didn't like it ❑
Couldn't make myself orgasm ❑
Don't think it's necessary ❑
Don't think it's important to do ❑
Don't care about it ❑
Rather do it with a partner ❑
Lack of privacy ❑
Other:

_____

_____

PLACES TO MASTURBATE

	Do it	Want to try	Maybe	No way
In my bed	❏	❏	❏	❏
In the bathroom/ shower/bathtub	❏	❏	❏	❏
In the car	❏	❏	❏	❏
At work	❏	❏	❏	❏
At the movies	❏	❏	❏	❏
In a hotel room	❏	❏	❏	❏

Other:

_____

_____

MY PREFERRED MASTURBATION ENVIRONMENT
Check off all that apply.

Music playing	❏	Favorite music?
No one home	❏	_____
Other people around	❏	
Bedtime	❏	
Morning	❏	
Fifteen-minute work break	❏	
Watching porn	❏	
Reading erotica/porn	❏	Favorite erotica/porn
Dark room	❏	_____
Fantasizing	❏	
Candles burning	❏	
Shades or curtains closed	❏	
Shades or curtains open	❏	
Quiet	❏	

Other:

_____

MASTURBATION TECHNIQUES (SEE PAGES 152–153
FOR MORE SPECIFIC DESCRIPTIONS OF THESE
TECHNIQUES)

	Do it	Want to try	Maybe	No way
Fist	❑	❑	❑	❑
Encircling the head	❑	❑	❑	❑
Five-finger	❑	❑	❑	❑
Three-finger	❑	❑	❑	❑
Backhand	❑	❑	❑	❑
Two hands	❑	❑	❑	❑
Slapping or whipping	❑	❑	❑	❑
Holding, rubbing, or jiggling testicles	❑	❑	❑	❑
Rubbing on or in a towel or pillow	❑	❑	❑	❑
Anal stimulation	❑	❑	❑	❑
Inserting between mattress and box spring	❑	❑	❑	❑
Inserting into a bag	❑	❑	❑	❑
Under running water	❑	❑	❑	❑
Using a condom with lube inside	❑	❑	❑	❑

Other:

SOUNDS I MAKE

	Always	Sometimes	Never	Maybe someday
No sound at all	❏	❏	❏	❏
Moan softly	❏	❏	❏	❏
Moan loudly	❏	❏	❏	❏
Have escalating moans	❏	❏	❏	❏
Breathe heavily	❏	❏	❏	❏
Pant	❏	❏	❏	❏
Scream	❏	❏	❏	❏
Cry	❏	❏	❏	❏
Laugh	❏	❏	❏	❏
Sing	❏	❏	❏	❏
Hold my breath	❏	❏	❏	❏
Call someone's name	❏	❏	❏	❏

Other:

_____

_____

MY MASTURBATION FANTASY

_____

_____

_____

_____

_____

What did you learn from doing this worksheet?

_____

_____

Chapter 9

A VISIT WITH YOUR LARGEST SEX ORGAN

Using Your Mind to Enhance Your Sexuality

* * *

When it comes to sex, our mind is probably the
most eager and athletic part of our anatomy.
It can dream, scheme, anticipate and remember.
—From Suzi Godson, *The Sex Book*

Minding Your Body

Picture this: Your senses are primed, blood is flowing to your genitals, you're feeling randy—you're on the road to one kick-ass sexual experience. Suddenly your partner mentions her "ex" and . . . all of your sexy feelings disappear. Why? Your brain, with all its complicated feelings and emotions, has stepped in to change the course of events.

Jimmy, thirty, recalls that *"in 1995 I was having sex with my girl-friend. The phone rang and I heard my brother leave a message on my*

answering machine telling me that Jerry Garcia had died. I was so up-
set I lost my erection and couldn't perform anymore."

So what can you do in such a situation? Well, as I see it, there
are two options: Accept the fact that you are no longer in the
mood and suggest that you two watch a movie or play a rousing
game of Scrabble, or suck it up, dive back in, and see if your
hormones can override the conflict going on in your mind.✭

As animalistic as humans can be, we are also rational, thinking emotional beings, which is why we read books about improving our sex lives instead of just fornicating like dogs in
heat. Your mind intensifies the experience of sex (but thinking
too much can sometimes do the opposite). Anatomically, many
areas of your brain are responsible for sexual arousal. The central region of your brain contains the *limbic system,* in which
the *amygdala* (no, not the Princess from *Star Wars*), *hypothalamus,*
and *septum* reside. The amygdala controls our emotional state
and affects how we interpret sexual stimuli. The hypothalamus
regulates sexual behavior, mediates how we feel pleasure, and
is involved with sexual and emotional expression. The septum is sometimes referred to as the "pleasure pathway" because
of its involvement with sexual pleasure. Your *cerebral cortex*, the
lumpy, bumpy layer of your brain (the gray matter) "matters"
in your ability to speak, to learn, to think, to perceive, and to
make choices. It is the home of sexual fantasies, daydreams, and
memories.

We cannot and should not completely separate our brains
from our genitals. No matter how young or old you are, your
mind is a terrible thing to waste.

✭ A word of caution: While it is normal to get turned off during sex
play from time to time, if this is happening regularly and if the slightest
distraction sends your erection packing or your clitoris into hiding, the
issue may be bigger than this book can address and you may want to
seek support from a licensed therapist.

Turn Me On

So what gets you going? People have preferences for certain partners, articles of clothing, body parts, skin color, foods, smells, settings, and behaviors. Most people know what turns them on, but they don't know why. You could spend ten years in therapy and still not have a clue why you go gaga for a guy with red pubes.

Kyla, twenty-four, says, *"The part of a man that turns me on the most is his hands. He has to have good hands that make it look like he works for a living. If he has small hands, then it makes him seem weak."*

You may have lust for someone at first sight or slowly develop a burning passion. What had once been an ardent affair may inexplicably fizzle out over time. Sometimes sexual chemistry is immediate:

"When I first met Darren, we just looked at each other and knew the sex was going to be great. The first time we slept together was mind-blowing and sustained us through a relationship that was pretty rocky in other ways." Allie, thirty-six.

On the other hand, sometimes chemistry takes a while to develop. But whether sustained or temporary, your attraction to others is based on a million different factors that can vary from time to time and place to place:

"I think I am attracted to different things in guys and girls. But one thing I am attracted to in both is confidence. Confidence really goes a long way!" Simone, twenty-eight.

"I was totally unattracted to my ex-boyfriend until the night we hooked up. He had been pursuing me for a while, and I just wasn't interested. But one night I saw him at a bar. He came up to me and said, 'We're going home together tonight.' I was totally turned off, but throughout the night he kept on coming over to me and saying that. Then at one point he leaned over and kissed me—and it was a really good kiss. At that point I went from being kind of grossed out to being

attracted to him. So, I said, 'Okay, let's go, it's now or never.' We went home together that night and then were together for quite a while, and it was all because he came up to me with confidence and told me we were going home together." Rebecca, twenty-eight.

"I had this crush on my eighth-grade science teacher, Miss Sharp. She was hot, in that 1970s kind of Farrah Fawcett way. I never missed earth science, and if she only knew how often I masturbated with her as the object of my lust!" Victor, forty-two.

"I had a big crush on my high school history teacher and used to try to spend as much time as possible with him. I volunteered to help him do office work after school one day a week. I was so crazy about him that I would get butterflies in my stomach on Mondays, knowing that I'd have him all to myself for an hour after school. I would always fantasize about him kissing me or falling in love with me. He was married and had two kids, but I was fifteen years old and not really thinking about that. One Monday after school, I was in his office and he came up behind me, put his arms around me, and told me that he thought I was very special. I was uncomfortable but didn't know what to say or do. He pulled me out of the chair and kissed me and told me that he loved me. I was nauseated but didn't say anything. I thought it was my fault, that I had brought it on because of my feelings for him. I think I was scared, unprepared, and stunned by the power of my 'feminine desires.' I never told my parents about it, and I stopped working for him after school and avoided talking to him in class. There was a huge gap between my fantasy of what I thought I wanted and the sleazy reality of what happened." Sheila, forty-six.

ACTIVITY: WHAT TURNS ME ON?

Use the following table to indicate what you find arousing. In the first column, "People," you can list specific people you know or celebrities, cartoon characters, historical figures, and so on. In the second column, "Places," list specific locations (such as Paris, the local diner, gas station bathrooms, parks), settings or scenarios, and the like that spark arousal. In the third column, "Things," record inanimate objects like clothing (bow ties, lace underwear), household items like tools and electronics, cars, music, books and other media, and so forth. For the final two columns, record personality traits (sense of humor, kind to animals, fearlessness . . .) and physical characteristics (love handles, red pubes, freckles . . .) that get you going.

People	Places	Things	Personality Traits	Physical Characteristics

A Trip to Fantasyland

Almost all of us fantasize at one point or another, and the type, frequency, and usage of our fantasies are limited only by our imagination. Anything goes when it's in your head; it's normal and healthy to fantasize. As Cathy Winks and Anne Semans write in *The Good Vibrations Guide to Sex,* "Fantasizing, like masturbating, is an act of self-love as well as an assertion of sexual confidence and independence. A creative fantasy life can contribute to a fulfilling, arousing sex life."

Using fantasy as inspiration, variation, and motivation for your sexploration. Maybe fantasy gets you horny and ready for your partner, or maybe you fantasize to help you get off with or without a partner. Your fantasies may be violent, kinky, fairy-tale-like, voyeuristic, action packed, comic, or tragic; they may involve past or current lovers, clergy, teachers, cartoon characters, same- or opposite-sex partners, multiple partners, total strangers, or farm animals. The most common fantasies involve having sex with someone other than your partner, forced encounters (being overpowered or "taken"), and watching or being watched. You can fantasize about having an affair, seducing a teacher, having your way with your favorite celebrity, or same-sex sessions.

Fantasies are portable; you can take them with you wherever you go. Time and place offer no barriers to what happens in your mind, so fantasize on the subway, at school, before going to sleep at night, in the shower, driving to work, at a meeting, instead of cleaning the car, or when shopping for groceries.

Some people have one reliable fantasy that always works for them; others create new ones that change constantly based on their current needs and desires. You can use your fantasies to enjoy sexual activities that you would never want to experience or to explore an alternate personality, sexual identity, or gender role.

Jamie, thirty-four, who is married and has two children, loves to fantasize about having sex with another woman: *"I would definitely say that I'm straight, but I find female bodies really attractive. When I get off, I fantasize about having another woman go down on me. I imagine that she would know exactly what I like and how I like it."*

Carlos, twenty-nine, says, *"Sometimes when I masturbate I use a butt plug and imagine I'm having sex with a guy from work. I don't think I'd ever really want to try anal sex with a guy, but I still like to think about it."*

Shawn, forty-one, who lives in Minnesota, is an avid runner. It's often bone-chillingly cold, and he runs bundled up and wearing a knit hat that covers most of his face: *"It looks like the kind of thing that a criminal wears in the movies. When I wear it I have this rape fantasy that totally turns me on. I would never rape anyone, but the fantasy is such a turn-on that I come home from running and keep my ski mask on while I masturbate."*

Isaac, who is eighty-five years old, has been getting *Playboy* since the early 1960s: *"I love reading the cartoons. My children tease me about it, and my daughter jokes that the centerfolds could be my great-grandchildren, but at least I'm still stimulated in my old age! They should be so lucky."*

Lisa, twenty-one, explains that she was never able to orgasm until she started fantasizing: *"I have to be totally in the fantasy in order to come. I usually like to think about being restrained or forced to pleasure multiple partners, and I can come only if I am totally lost in the fantasy."*

"I had these great rescue fantasies as a kid," recalls Maria, forty-six. *"They featured Batman and Robin and how they saved me from all kinds of perilous situations. Even now my fantasies involve being rescued, emotionally or physically, by the man of my dreams. It's that knight in shining armor who's coming any day now. Yeah, right."*

Wanda, thirty-six, says, *"In real life I totally make fun of romance novels. But sometimes when my boyfriend is going down on me, I imagine I am a nineteenth-century heiress who has been kidnapped and forced to be the sex slave of some Fabio-looking guy. I would never date a dude with a mullet in real life, and I would never tell my boyfriend what I was imagining. Oh my God, he would never go down on me again!"*

Fantasyland Attractions: Role-Play

Role-play can be a great way to act out your fantasies, give yourself an opportunity to take a vacation from yourself by pretending that you're somebody else (cheerleader, military leader, German in *lederhosen*, whatever), or invigorate your relationship. You may experiment with role-play one afternoon and end up laughing hysterically or take role-play very seriously and use it as an integral part of your personal life.

Dressing up or down can decrease your inhibition for new sexual adventures. Of course, not all of us are comfortable in or turned on by a corset, stiletto heels, fishnet stockings, or a red leather jock strap, but even a small change (from boxers to briefs) may be enough to kindle desire. Adding props like a feather duster, teddy bear, stethoscope, or latex gloves (yes, Doctor, I'm ready for my prostate exam!) can add stimulation and sensation to any activity.

Here are some comments from others:

"When I got married, I got all of this sexy lingerie as shower gifts. It was so not me. I tried to wear it to turn my husband on, but I always felt silly. He said he was much more turned on when I would wear a white tank top and my Hello Kitty boy-cut underwear." SuJin, twenty-six.

"I told my boyfriend that I was getting him a massage for his birthday and that the massage therapist was coming to his house. When the time came, I put on a wig and dressed up as the masseuse and rang his doorbell. When he answered the door, I introduced myself as Charlene and said that his girlfriend had hired me as a birthday treat. He wasn't totally sure what was going on, but he played along. It was amazing. I gave him a massage and was so turned on. Being in costume and pretending freed me up to do stuff I never would have done otherwise.

When it was over, he told me it was the best massage he'd ever had and that he hoped his girlfriend would hire me again soon." Shakira, thirty-one.

"My ex-girlfriend and I once videotaped ourselves having sex. It had always been one of my fantasies to be in a porn film. It was so liberating, we really got into it once the initial shyness wore off. Performing for the camera allowed us to do all kinds of kinky stuff we normally never did. Watching it was a trip. Then we destroyed it because we're both teachers and would lose our jobs if anyone saw it." Randall, forty-four.

"My friend Jean and I used to play this game. It was called 'movie star.' During movie star we would play a mother-daughter duo who were fallen movie stars. The reason for our fall? The mean male boss had 'violated' us in some way and thrown us out on the street. Neither of us knew the word rape *at the time, but I sometimes think of this as a really early rape fantasy/role-play."* Tessa, twenty-six.

"I like a woman who lets you talk about your fantasies and how to make them better. If you tell a woman your fantasy when you are out with her and she wants to go into the bathroom and talk about it a little more—that's the right reaction!" Robin, thirty-two.

Many a traveler has come back with tales of vacation sexploits that make life at home seem, well, positively dull. As my usually reserved friend Maya says proudly, "I got driven out of Peru because I slept with all of the men there!" Now, sleeping with an entire country may not exactly be your cup of tea, but there are other ways to be adventurous that don't necessarily mean dropping your pants thirty times a day.

"I went to Club Med with a co-worker and for the first time in my life understood why sororities are popular! We seriously turned on sorority girl party mode, danced with our shirts off, flirted with everyone we met, made out with each other in public, and generally had a kick-ass time. I am always pretty reserved and have had sex with only one person, and that was a long time ago, so it was a really different side of me.

My co-worker and I are still cool, though we've never tried to relive that here!" Nattie, twenty-seven.

Creative Inspiration

Just as with any creative endeavor, you may need inspiration for fantasy from time to time. Creative fantasy ideas are available from your dreams, your past experiences, romance novels, straight or gay erotica, movies, Web logs—really from anywhere.

Jack Morin, in his recommended book *The Erotic Mind,* claims that understanding our peak sexual experiences and fantasies offers the greatest opportunity for self-discovery and, consequently, revitalized sexual experiences. He discusses how anxiety, guilt, and anger, generally thought to have a negative impact on sexual arousal, often turn out to be aphrodisiacs and why dynamic and risky is usually more arousing than static and safe.

One possible issue with using erotica or porn for fantasy is that some of the images may be disturbing or degrading and, because they are staged and acted, may set up unrealistic expectations. Keep in mind that fantasy is not reality, that you don't need to emulate what you see, and that part of sexploration is discovering what turns you off as well as what turns you on. If you are sharing your erotica or porn with another person as a way to get turned on, be sure that what you are using is seductive to all parties involved. Enjoy the following turn-on stories:

"My freshman year of college, we used to gather at night and read the letters in Penthouse *that would describe random sexual encounters with pool boys, deliverymen, flight attendants, etc. We would argue about whether they were real-life adventures or made-up tales written by drunk fraternity boys. Either way, they sparked my imagination."* Jonathon, twenty-nine.

"I think I was about twelve years old and in summer camp when I first heard about pages 26 and 27 of The Godfather. *The girls in my bunk*

would giggle about it, but I hadn't read it. So when I came home at the end of the summer, I went straight to my parents' bookshelves and took it. Turns out that it's a pretty graphic scene where Sonny has sex with some bridesmaid at a wedding and there's stickiness between her legs. Didn't really turn me on, but it did get me wondering." Becca, thirty-six.

"Masturbating to images of Betty Dodson teaching women how to have orgasms in a video that I bought really helps me with my lesbian fantasies." Cerisse, twenty-seven.

"Porn? It's stupid and boring. All I can think about is the actors being strung out on drugs, getting HIV, not being into it." Tyrone, fifty.

"My uncle worked for Playboy," writes Sari, twenty-four, who identifies as bisexual, *"and the first time I flipped through the pages of a Playboy I was probably only about five years old. My cousin took me into the bathroom at her house and excitedly showed me the shocking pictures of naked women. We locked the door and admired the beautiful bodies we hoped to grow into one day. I think it was a very positive way for us to explore, and I think it helped to further my curiosity about porn in general. When I was about ten, I started sneaking into my brother's room to search for porn, and when I found some, I was brave enough to steal it for weeks at a time for my own use. Ultimately, I think these positive childhood experiences with porn really allowed me to explore some of the questions I had at the time. Pornography really affected my sexuality in a positive way as I was growing up, and as I'm older I still feel that it is a positive, healthy aspect of my sexuality today."*

MY FANTASY WORKSHEET

Here are some "basic" fantasies that are frequently cited in books, videos, and other erotic venues. For each one, place an X in the appropriate column to indicate how you feel about it. In the last two columns, indicate whether it would be for your mind only or whether you could see yourself actually acting it out with someone else. There's also room for you to write in other scenarios based on what you like.

	Love it!	Maybe	Nope, not for me	Yuck!	Would want to role-play	For my mind only!
Being overpowered or "taken"						
Being disciplined by teacher or other authority figure						
Watching others						
Being watched; having sex in a public place						
Celebrity or other famous person						
Bondage or sado-masochism						
Taboo or illegal adventure						
Changing sexual orientation						
Multiple partners or group sex						

	Love it!	Maybe	Nope, not for me	Yuck!	Would want to role-play	For my mind only!
Anonymous sex						
Cybersex or phone sex						
Someone who is not your current partner, but someone you know						
Different ethnicity or nationality						
Vacation or other travel adventure						

Select one of the basic fantasies above that gets you turned on and write a story with more detail and embellishment. Think about the time, place, season, person(s) involved, clothing, props, and so on that you would need to fully describe what happens. Remember, it's a fantasy, so anything goes! Write the description on a separate piece of paper.

Pick a fantasy that you would want to role-play with someone else. What would get in the way of your being able to role-play this fantasy with a partner?

_____

_____

_____

How might you deal with the barriers that you listed above?

_____

_____

_____

CONCERNS ABOUT FANTASIES*

Many of us have an unwritten code about what is appropriate material for fantasy. When our imaginations cross the line, we might feel guilt or fear that something's wrong with us. Here are some common anxieties people experience when it comes to fantasy:

- Some people feel guilty if their fantasies do not involve their current partners, but fantasizing about someone else doesn't necessarily mean your partner is dispensable or any less desirable. If your partner is giving you grief about fantasizing about someone else, try explaining that your fantasy isn't an indication that you want someone else, it simply increases your sexual excitement, which benefits you both.
- People fear that if they are fantasizing about some taboo-breaking activity, they must harbor a secret desire to actually do it. Taboo subject matter is infused with erotic significance almost by definition. The forbidden, the mysterious, and the dangerous have a seductive appeal. There is absolutely no indication that having a fantasy automatically leads to acting on that fantasy.

- There are no standards for how much someone should fantasize, so there is no "too much" or "too little" fantasizing. The only barometer is if your fantasies interfere with your ability to function daily—then you may want to seek professional help.
- If you're unable to accept your fantasies (for instance, if your thoughts are dominated by an abusive ex-lover), or if they exacerbate a sense of low self-esteem or self-hatred, you can take steps to change your pattern by discovering new arousing images to supplant old ones.

*Adapted from *The Good Vibrations Guide to Sex*
by Cathy Winks and Anne Semans

Chapter 10

PLEASURE ISLAND

Trips to Erotic Lands

✳ ✳ ✳

Kama Sutra everyone!!
—From *Hair*

*D*on't you find it gratifying when you are really into what you are doing, whether it's jogging in the park, playing poker, reading a good mystery novel, watching someone open birthday presents, or sucking on your lover's earlobe? Isn't it great, too, when another person is sharing the experience, vigorously absorbed and energized by what is happening, so that it's mutually synergistic? Wouldn't you enjoy it less if you were critiquing every moment of it or judging your performance? How do you allow yourself to sink into sybaritic pleasurable sensations rather than wallowing in intellectual thoughts or sexual self-criticism? What gets in the way?

Greer, thirty-four, says, *"Here's the message I got from my parents: Sex is dirty, so you should save yourself for the one you love. What the hell is that supposed to mean? I should save doing something dirty for the person I love? Then it will be a beautiful experience?! Yeah, that makes so much sense. No wonder we're all confused about sex."*

"Sex and pleasure were not mentioned in the same sentence in my house," recalls Norma, sixty-two. *"My mom told me that sex was something you did after you got married and it was your obligation to do it even if you didn't enjoy it. I doubt that she ever enjoyed sex; I doubt she ever even knew that she was capable of enjoying sex."*

Jennifer, forty-three, learned positive lessons about sensuality from her mom: *"My mom was very tactile. She loved the feel of pussy willows against her cheek, a fur collar around her neck, and she collected Lalique glass because she loved how smooth it felt when she touched it. There was this one piece, a glass platter that was frosted on the top. I remember it so clearly because every time she used it, she would call it her 'penis glass' plate and run her hand over its smooth surface. I didn't really understand what she meant. It wasn't until I got older and had touched a few penises myself that I realized that the glass platter did feel exactly like the soft, smooth skin on the head of a penis! She had died by then, so I never got to share with her how that image had stayed with me all of those years."*

Zane, twenty-six, says, *"The position of 69 is just surreal—69 is an exotic and purely indulgent position for a couple because there is no intercourse. The sex is so intimate because of the senses involved. The smell and taste are heightened along with the sight, the touch, and the sounds. I think people pleasuring people are the luckiest people in the world!"*

Tamara Kreinin, president of SIECUS, sums it up this way: *"We keep pleasure as the ultimate secret of sexuality yet assume that when they are old enough (and in a relationship that is approved of) all people will be able to have it."*★

★ From *Sexual Pleasure*. SIECUS Report 30, no. 4 (April/May 2002).

EXERCISE

Think back about the messages you received from family, peers, religious institutions, and others about sexual pleasure. What do you recall? What messages have you gotten in your life about sex and pleasure? How has sexual pleasure been described for you?

_____

_____

_____

How would you describe your personal philosophy about sexual pleasure?

_____

_____

_____

In the Realm of the Senses

One of the best parts of traveling is experiencing new sights, smells, and tastes. I remember going to the island of Santorini for the first time and the exhilaration I felt seeing row after row of pristine white houses with vibrant blue doors dotting the mountainside. It was visual ecstasy.

You may feel strong visceral reactions to the taste of homemade pie, the feel of newly washed bedsheets against your skin, or the sound of rain against your tent. There is sensuality in everything you see, feel, touch, taste, and smell. "When we are born our senses are already formed. But as we grow, our senses form us. They are our antennae, our awareness, our instinct, the way we meet the world and the way the world meets us," writes Suzi Godson in *The Sex Book*.

SEXERCISE: CHOOSING WHAT PLEASES YOU

If you already know how to make yourself feel good through self-pleasuring, then theoretically sex with a partner could feel that good, too. Often what holds us back are concerns about what our partner would think if we were to offer suggestions and express our needs and desires (whether sexual, emotional, or physical). Therefore, instead of "Oh wow, that feels good, oh yeah, oh yeah," what goes through our mind is, "That would feel so much better if it were just a bit to the right," or, "God, I wish he'd kept doing that," or, "I feel so alone in this relationship, it's as though I'm not even here," and so on. I believe that most people like to see their partners relish pleasure and would try (within reason) to fulfill their wishes.

One skill that may help you feel more sexually nurtured is to be able to control how someone else pleases you. Putting up with something that doesn't feel good just because you're hoping it will be over soon is not helpful or pleasurable and can reinforce negative feelings about your sexuality. For this exercise, you will need a sexual partner. If this partner is someone with whom you have an ongoing relationship, tell him or her that you're trying to undo some unhelpful habits, and ask if he or she would be willing to make love to you with the understanding that you're going to speak up *every time* you can think of a way in which what is happening could feel better to you.

If you are getting together with a new partner for the first time, one way to take some of the pressure off your uncertainty about each other's likes and dislikes is to say, "Mmmm, I want you to have a really good time tonight. While I'm getting to know what you like, just let me know any time you can think of a way what we're doing could feel better and I'll do the same for you."

When pleasuring a partner, try to get inside his or her head and imagine what he or she would like. As you gain experience with this person, you can eventually learn what he or she likes (everyone is a little different, after all). The ultimate goal is to be able to key your arousal into your partner's, so the more turned on your partner gets the more turned on you get. You can reach this place by imagining you are experiencing whatever you are doing to him or her.

For most men and women, arousal begins when they receive some type of sexual stimulation: a touch, smell, sight, thought, or anything that has erotic meaning for them. Clearly, our five senses play a crucial role in pleasurable sexual experiences.

Touch

T-t-t-touch me, I wanna be touched," sings Susan Sarandon in the movie *Rocky Horror Picture Show.* She is craving touch, and that's understandable because touch is quite potent and powerful.

Touch is so important that infants who are not held or touched may suffer from what is called "failure to thrive," a condition that can lead to their death. Aline P. Zoldbrod, in her wise and warm book *Sex Smart,* writes that "touch is the foundation upon which your ability to enjoy sexuality is built; it is vital to loving and to sexual expression."

Your skin is a sensory organ with nerve endings that respond to touch, pressure, and temperature changes. Some parts of your body have more nerve endings than others (for instance, your clitoris, nipples, lips, fingertips, and genitals), and these areas are more responsive to touch. People love different sensations on their bodies. Some people like to be caressed lightly. Others need a firm grip. Some want only to be hugged, while others need concentration just on the genitals.

Kim, forty-five, explains, *"I got into the [BDSM] scene in my thirties. For me it is not as much about being restrained as it is about being spanked. I need to have that intense feeling. I also have various piercings, nipples, clit hood, partly because I love the way it feels when they are tugged on and I think they look great, but I also appreciate the actual experience of getting pierced. For me it is all about how things feel, and the more intense the feeling, the better for me an experience is."*

Nicole, thirty-six, says, *"I love having my elbows rubbed with lotion. I have had a partner call them my 'elbow clits.' "*

One way to explore touch is to experiment with sensation play. Try taking a feather duster, Brillo pad, stuffed animal, or other item and trailing it over different parts of your body without touching your genitals. Notice the sensations that you feel as you vary the textures and pressure of the objects on different body parts. There are so many places on the human body that feel amazing when touched, try not to focus all your attention on the few obvious spots. Yes, the breasts, nipples, buttocks, penis, and vulva are sexy places to touch. We also see images of people going gaga over having their neck caressed, but aside from these few places, much of the body is overlooked when it comes to sensual touch.

ACTIVITY: THINGS TO TOUCH, WAYS TO TOUCH

One way to expand your sexual pleasure is to expand your creativity. The following exercise will help you think about different methods for doing basic activities. It called "Things to Touch, Ways to Touch." You can do it solo or make it a game for two or more. Variations on this exercise include "Things to Lick, Ways to Lick," "Things to Suck, Ways to Suck," "Things to Penetrate, Ways to Penetrate," and so on!

Instructions: Each of us likes to be touched in different places and in different ways. Fill in the blanks in the following chart to help you figure out how and where you might like to be touched and in what way. You might have touched a lot of these places in the course of your everyday life, washing, dressing, and so on, but for this exercise try to think about these body parts as potential sources of pleasure rather than as places you need to shave.

Check the boxes (more than one may apply) to indicate which parts of your body you like or do not like to have touched intimately. Feel free to be more explicit in your descriptions:

Body Part	Yes!	Maybe	No way	Would touch myself, but not let someone else touch this	Would let a partner touch, but wouldn't touch my own	Would touch myself and would let a partner touch
Cheeks						
Eyes						
Lips						
Inside mouth						
Inside ear						
Top of head						
Hair						
Earlobe						
Neck (what part?)						
Shoulders						
Breasts						
Chest						
Nipples						
Underarms						
Arms						

Body Part	Yes!	Maybe	No way	Would touch myself, but not let someone else touch this	Would let a partner touch, but wouldn't touch my own	Would touch myself and would let a partner touch
Hands						
Fingers						
Stomach						
Belly button						
Inner thighs						
Outer thighs						
Labia						
Mons pubis						
Clitoris						
Vagina						
Penis glans						
Penis shaft						
Scrotum						
Perineum						
Anus						

Body Part	Yes!	Maybe	No way	Would touch myself, but not let someone else touch this	Would let a partner touch, but wouldn't touch my own	Would touch myself and would let a partner touch
Buttocks						
Calves						
Knees						
Feet						
Toes						
Other						

Now, for parts that you enjoy having touched, check off the boxes for ways in which you would like having those parts touched:

Body part	With fingers	Tongue or mouth	With feet	Partner's genitals	With sex toy	With ice	With feather	Breath	Other
Cheeks									
Eyes									
Lips									
Inside mouth									
Inside ear									
Top of head									
Hair									
Earlobe									
Neck (what part?)									
Shoulders									
Breasts									
Chest									

Body part	With fingers	Tongue or mouth	With feet	Partner's genitals	With sex toy	With ice	With feather	Breath	Other
Nipples									
Underarms									
Arms									
Hands									
Fingers									
Stomach									
Belly button									
Inner thighs									
Outer thighs									
Labia									
Mons pubis									
Clitoris									
Vagina									
Penis glans									
Penis shaft									

Body part	With fingers	Tongue or mouth	With feet	Partner's genitals	With sex toy	With ice	With feather	Breath	Other
Scrotum									
Perineum									
Anus									
Buttocks									
Calves									
Knees									
Feet									
Toes									
Other									

Now think about how you would like those parts touched:

Body part	Softly	Firmly	Intense pressure	Teasingly	Circular motion	Nibble	Tickle	Stop and go	Other
Face									
Eyes									
Lips									
Mouth									
Cheeks									
Ears									
Head/hair									
Neck (what part?)									
Shoulders									
Breasts									
Chest									
Nipples									
Underarms									
Arms									

Body part	Softly	Firmly	Intense pressure	Teasingly	Circular motion	Nibble	Tickle	Stop and go	Other
Hands									
Stomach									
Belly button									
Inner thighs									
Outer thighs									
Vulva (Labia and Mons)									
Clitoris									
Vagina									
Penis									
Scrotum									
Perineum									
Anus									
Buttocks									
Calves									
Other									

Here are some other words to describe other types of touch you might want to explore:

- Caress
- Stroke
- Fondle
- Massage
- Rub
- Spank
- Smack
- Hug
- Pat
- Embrace
- Cuddle
- Knead
- Slap
- Tap
- Hold
- Paw
- Snuggle
- Pet
- Work
- Squeeze
- Nuzzle

And here are some more words to describe ways you might want someone to do that:

- Gentle
- Rough
- Tender
- Forceful
- Soft
- Hard
- Light
- Firm

See if you can come up with some more:

_____   _____   _____   _____   _____

You might want to be even more specific in your description. For example, a tongue can be used in many ways: probe with the tip of the tongue, lick with the top of the tongue, swaddle with the underside of the tongue.

Think about how you might want to tell a partner to touch you. Combine the previous charts to create your request:

- Honey, it would get me really excited if you teased my inner thighs gently with the tip of your tongue in a circular motion.
- I'd love it if you massaged my feet firmly with your thumbs.
- Please spank my butt rapidly with that stuffed bunny. Start lightly but build up in intensity until I tell you to stop.
- Would you mind rubbing your penis slowly around the perimeter of my face?

Now it's your turn! Create as many as you'd like.

_____

_____

_____

_____

Tasty De-lights

𝒰mm, yumm, delish! That's right; the human body can be a tasty, tasty thing. Adults have about ten thousand taste buds, so how your partner tastes when you kiss him or her can be an important factor. Savor how your partner's skin, body fluids, or breath tastes.

Here are a few comments about taste:

"I loved it when Marcus would climb into bed without showering.

His skin always had this salty, musky taste to it. I never wanted to tell him because I thought he would think I was gross, but I really liked it." Alex, twenty-one.

"I had a girlfriend once who was really uncomfortable with oral sex. She would insist on douching before every time. It really changed the experience. I didn't want to taste a rose, I wanted to taste her. We were together for ages, but I can't really tell you what she actually tasted like." Patsy, forty-one.

"When a woman enjoys the taste of her own vagina after experiencing an orgasm on the face of her lover, that is absolutely the hottest thing in the world." Mark, thirty-eight.

Some women are terrified that their vulvas taste bad. But unless a woman has a vaginal infection, this is not usually an issue. However, smoking, alcohol, medication, and diet can affect the way someone tastes. If you do not enjoy the taste of a vulva, you can always use a latex dam or square of plastic wrap for oral sex.

The same thing holds true for men. Men have been known to alter their diets in search of delicious-tasting semen. *"I read somewhere that drinking grapefruit made your cum taste better,"* says Jerome, thirty-four. *"So I tried it for a while. I think it did make a difference. It seemed a lot sweeter and less bitter."*

If you don't find semen to be seemly, you can ask your partner to ejaculate outside of your mouth or use a condom.

Your body is the perfect slate for embellishing with tasty treats. "Eat me" has an entirely different connotation when you're talking about covering the body with any number of sauces and garnishes. Everything tastes better with skin!

"My husband loves the candy Circus Peanuts. One night I put them all over my body (they stick on skin if you lick the back of them first), and he ate them off of me. Now he gets hard when he sees a bag of them." Heather, forty-eight.

"When I was in college, my first girlfriend and I were working our way through The Joy of Sex, *trying everything. There was this stuff*

called *Magic Shell*, which formed a hard chocolate crust when you poured it over ice cream, and we decided it would be cool to pour Magic Shell on my penis so that she could nibble on a chocolate-shelled dick. When she poured it on, it just stayed a gross, goopy liquid. At first we couldn't figure out what went wrong, but then we realized that ice cream is frozen and cold and my dick was warm, so the shell wasn't ever going to form. We tried rubbing ice cubes on my dick, but it didn't work and we were just making a big mess. It was fun, though." David, fifty.

"My partner and I were celebrating a promotion he'd gotten at work and were toasting with a lovely red wine. Trying to be creative, I stuck my penis in the wine, thinking it would be erotic if he could lick it off. It burned like hell! My advice—don't put alcohol in your urethra." Kim, forty-two.

ACTIVITY: MY TASTY TURN-ONS AND -OFFS

Think about what tastes you enjoy and what tastes turn you off—consider body flavors and beyond. Here is a list to get you started; use these or create your own.

	Yummy	Yucky	Maybe, under these conditions...
Chocolate			
Semen			
Vaginal fluids			

	Yummy	Yucky	Maybe, under these conditions....
Garlic			
Sweat			
Coffee			
Jelly			
Lips			

Follow Your Nose

𝓗umans, like animals, produce sex smells called *pheromones* that are designed to attract partners. Several years ago, a study was done where a number of married women applied a drop or two of their vaginal discharge to their chests before they went to bed at night. A control group was used whose members applied nothing. The results: The husbands of the appliers initiated sex much more frequently than did the other husbands!

Smells play a significant role in arousal. In the Western world, we dedicate time, energy, and financial resources to eradicating body odor, but in other cultures body odors are considered incredibly sexy. This may actually be affecting our sex lives more than we know. As Rick, twenty-nine, says, *"I don't expect sex to be totally clean—that's what showers are for. I love it when the room gets all funky from all the fucking."*

"I love that sweaty outdoor smell that my boyfriend has after he's played his middle-aged Sunday-in-the-park football game." Simon, thirty-five.

"There's something about the smell of beer and cigarettes that's a real turn-on for me. It smells like my rebellious teenage years when I was making out in bars and breaking curfew. It brings out the 'bad girl' sexy part of me." Connie, thirty-eight.

Of course, there's a difference between turn-on odors and turn-off odors:

"I was dating this guy I was attracted to, but he also had a girlfriend at another school, and they were having sex, so he didn't want to have it with me, too. After wearing down his resolve (I can be rather persistent), he agreed. When he arrived for the big event, he reeked of garlic— I swear, he must've eaten an entire head of it. The sex was fine, but I kept holding my breath because he smelled so bad. That was nineteen years ago, and to this day, I can't have sex with or kiss anyone who has garlic breath." Wendy, forty-one.

ACTIVITY: WHAT MY NOSE KNOWS

Think about what smells you enjoy and what smells turn you off—consider body odors and beyond. Here is a list to get you started; use these or create your own.

	Mmm!	Ew!	Maybe, under these conditions . . .
Cookies baking			
Vulva			
Neck			
Garlic			
Sweaty skin			
Flowers (any specific ones?)			
Freshly cut grass			
Perfume or aftershave (specify)			
Ivory soap			

Sightseeing

𝒪ne of those "Mercury-Uranus" myths is that men are turned on by visuals, but women are turned on by romance. That's nonsense! Both men and women get turned on by looking at things they find sexy, including each other:

"One of my lovers used to be fascinated by the part of my breast that curved under my armpit. He loved to look at it and said that it was one of the sexiest parts of my body." Heidi, fifty-nine.

"I love watching my boyfriend sleep. I get to stare at every part of his body without having to be concerned about him looking back or feeling weird that I'm staring at him." Guy, thirty-eight.

"The sight of my lover can literally make me weak in my knees. I always thought that was a cliché, but it's true! Just seeing her face, my heart skips a beat and I get butterflies in my stomach and my legs are wobbly. I'm a damn cliché of lust." Pissaro, twenty-nine.

For some, being able to watch during sex, particularly with the lights on, makes an encounter more enjoyable and intimate. But that can be challenging for people who are insecure about how they look naked or uncomfortable with seeing themselves tangled up in some crazy position. Keep in mind that most people who enjoy watching what is happening while they have sex probably aren't counting your wrinkles or noticing your butt rash. Interestly, attraction causes our eyes to widen and pupils to dilate, while lust causes our eyes to narrow and become less focused (e.g., bedroom eyes). Here are descriptions of what some people like to watch:

"I love lying in bed and watching my lady get undressed. Even if she isn't trying to be sexy, seeing her take off different pieces of clothing and then her underwear always gets me in the mood for sex." Jermaine, thirty-nine.

"My boyfriend always wants to keep the lights on during sex. I'm kind of shy, so we compromise and light candles. That way he can still see what is going on, but I don't feel as exposed." Francie, eighteen.

ACTIVITY: I SEE

Think about what images you enjoy seeing, what sights turn you on and which ones turn you off—consider body parts and beyond. Here is a list to get you started; use these or create your own.

	A sight for sore eyes	Get my blindfold	Maybe, under these conditions . . .
Erotic art			
Vulva			
Buttocks			
Same-sex images			
Sexually explicit images (specify)			
Breasts			
Erect penis			

Aural Sex

ℋearing is an often underrated sense when it comes to sex. Ever wonder why there are so many phone sex hot lines out there? Hearing someone talk about sex and listening to the sounds that person makes during sexual encounters (heavy breathing, whispers, giggles, and moans) can really up the sexual ante.

Some people like sex talk dirty and crave hearing things like "Fuck my pussy, you raging hard-on of a man." Others like their talk slow and sweet and dotted with praise ("Oh baby, you touch me so good") and declarations of emotion. A lot of people like a little bit of both. Of course, our partners can't know that nothing makes your erection disappear faster than hearing the word *hump* or nothing gets you hotter than having "Drop trou and go for it" whispered in your ear. Talk doesn't even have to be about sex to work for you. It can be a real turn-on to hear how smart or talented you are, what a great butt you have, or how your partner really digs the heart you shaved into your pubic hair.

Another aspect of aural sex is the sounds that emanate from your body during sexual encounters. One of the most potentially embarrassing sounds is the vaginal fart, which I like to call a "vart." A vart is the product of air being pushed into the vagina during repeated penetration. This is normal and natural and can be an opportunity for some hot hilarity. Varts are not gas, but farting can also be a by-product of sexual activity. Holding it in can be distracting, but letting it out (especially if it's one of those "silent but deadly" types) can be distracting, too. Sometimes you just have no choice.

Then there are the sounds that we make during sex. Are you a screamer? A moaner? An "I'm having a religious experience—thank you, Lord, thank you!" person? Maybe you are more of a squeaker (eek!) or the silent, self-contained type. Do you laugh or cry after you come? These are all normal sexual reactions, and for some, hearing the sounds that erupt from their partner makes the experience much more erotic:

"I love it when I hear my boyfriend's breathing getting more intense and I can tell he is about to come. It makes me even hornier." Ken, twenty-six.

"My wife makes these incredible moans when I hit her hot spots. Just thinking about it gets me hard." John, thirty-two.

"After I come, I always laugh. I used to be embarrassed about it, because I was afraid that the person I was with would think I was laughing at him or her, but now I just tell them it's the joy of the release, the joy of being alive, the joy of sharing my body with another person. I only laugh if I come with another person, though, not if I masturbate." Suzy, fifty-three.

Last, there is the sound of music (Baron von Trapp fantasy, anyone?). Music can set the mood, rev you up, turn you on, calm you down, and/or convey a potent message. Sensual music connoisseurs sing the praises of Luther Vandross and swear by the seductive crooning of Frank Sinatra, but you may have your own particular artist whose talented trilling titillates you time after time. Enjoy boffing to Beethoven? Getting randy to rap? Prefer punk rock passion?

"Led Zeppelin became my big make-out music in high school. Whenever a Zeppelin song comes on the radio and I hear the first few notes, I get all juicy." Jasmine, thirty-four.

ACTIVITY: AURAL AROUSALS

	Turn up the volume	Put it on mute	Maybe, under these conditions . . .
My lover's moans			
Music (specify)			
Heavy breathing			
Sex talk (specify)			
My name			
Whispered words (specify)			
Slurping			
Lips			

REFLECTION

Think about your sexual experiences, either solo or with a partner.

Which sense seems to be most important to you in those experiences?

Taste ❑
Touch ❑
Sound ❑
Smell ❑
Sight ❑

Why do you think that is?
_____
_____

Which sense seems to be least important to you?
Taste ❑
Touch ❑
Sound ❑
Smell ❑
Sight ❑

Why do you think that is?
_____
_____

Which sense would you most like to explore? How do you think you could enhance your sensory experiences for the one you have chosen?
_____
_____

Variety Is the Spice of Life

*B*ut what if your senses are honed, you totally love your body, you feel connected with your partner, and you're still looking to shake things up? Rest assured, even the most seasoned sex

LUBRICANTS: SENSORY ENHANCERS

Face it, sex is gooey. There is sweat and semen and saliva and all kinds of other slippery and slide-y sensational secretions. That's what makes it fun. But let's say you find yourself in one of the following situations:

- You just aren't as juicy as you'd like to be (could be hormones, medication, end of a randy weekend).
- You want even more juicy goodness than you have.
- You're about to try something new, like anal penetration, that requires lots of juice.

What can you do? Bring on the lubricant. Not all lubes are created equal, however. They differ in their chemical makeup, their thickness, their texture, their taste, the amount of time they last, and their compatibility with specific activities and items.

Here are some lube basics for you:

- Oil-based lubricants such as canola, corn, or coconut oil or baby oil should *never* be used with latex barriers like condoms because oil destroys latex! Use water-based lubes with latex.
- Oil-based lubes are great for masturbating a penis, but they should never be used inside a vagina.
- Anything that goes into the vagina needs an unscented water-based lubricant. You can always reactivate a water-based lubricant by adding a few drops of water or some saliva. Women who are prone to yeast infections should avoid lubes that contain glycerin. Lubricants that contain nonoxynol-9 (a spermicide) may cause vaginal irritation and increase risk of infection.
- Silicone lubes feel like oil but are water based, so you can use them with latex condoms and dental dams. For those who like to

have sex in bathtubs, hot tubs, and other watery venues, silicone lube is great since it washes off more slowly than other lubes.

• Silicone lubricant should *not* be used on silicone sex toys. The silicone in the lube gradually dissolves the silicone in the sex toy. You can solve this problem by covering your silicone sex toy first with a latex condom (it also makes cleanup so much easier!).

For more comprehensive information about lubrication, check out www.babeland.com and www.goofyfootpress.com/menu.html.

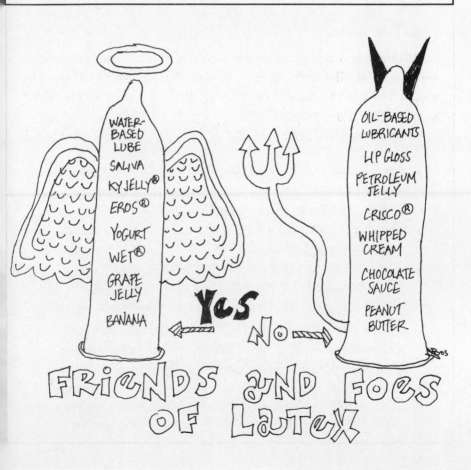

veterans sometimes need a change. Some folks find that if they
have fallen into a bit of a sex rut, trying new sexual activities
can be a great kick start. This doesn't mean that you should
join the mile-high club if you hate flying. It might mean something as simple as having sex with the lights on if you are a
lights off–er. Or trying out a new location (just don't get arrested for public indecency and blame it on this book).

Some people always have sex at night, but morning sex or
even an afternoon delight can add a bit of diversity to your typical sex routine. Change doesn't have to mean you pierce your
tongue, put on crotchless underwear, and expect miracles. There
are a million ways to spice things up that you might not even realize you could do.

- Does your partner always initiate sex? Why don't you
  try initiating sex for a change and see what happens.
- Has your sexual routine become, well, routine? Is it
  always the same old, same old—kissing, then oral sex,
  then intercourse, then sleep? Try having intercourse
  before oral sex. It's a cheap, simple, and surefire way
  to shake things up.
- Change positions. This doesn't mean you have to
  break your back trying out contortions that even yoga
  aficionados like Madonna can't master, but if you are
  usually on top, get on the bottom. Used to doing it
  from behind? Why not mix it up and shift to the side?
- How about introducing a toy? Sex toys do not have
  to be big, scary dildos. A lot of toys are simple
  massagers and ticklers, designed more for sensation
  than penetration (see "Toyland," page 226, for more
  about toys).
- What about adding some lubricant to the mix? Lube
  now comes in flavors, colors, and even a special heat-
  up variety.

- And, yes, you knew it was coming . . . erotica! A lot of people are shy about introducing erotica into the bedroom (or at this point in your sexploration, the kitchen, dining room, or backyard), but erotic images, films, or books can add a new element to the sex lives of even the most adventurous couples.

Backdoor Basics

𝒟o you have an anus? If so, you are a candidate for anal eroticism. Anal taboos (it's dirty; it's an out-hole, not an in-hole) inhibit most people from thinking, talking, and learning about the sexual use of the anus, but millions of men and women, straight, gay, and bisexual, experiment with anal sex. Thirty-five years ago, Kinsey stated that the anal region had erotic significance for about half of the population. In one more recent survey, 47 percent of men and 61 percent of women admitted to having tried anal intercourse.

The anal taboo can be thrilling and a source of "dirty," sleazy, forbidden excitement. Rimming enthusiasts may enjoy the feeling that they are being disgustingly—and delightfully—perverse. Other people regard the anus as a secret, special place. Sharing it with a partner is an act of openness and giving.

There are many ways to enjoy anal eroticism, including fingering your anus while masturbating or stimulating your partner's anus during intercourse or oral sex, gently inserting and rotating a finger during sex play, or using a dildo or vibrator for sensation or insertion. Some people enjoy the feelings of pressure and fullness that insertion provides, especially once they understand that this sensation does not mean that they are going to have a bowel movement.

The anus is rife with nerve endings, most of them around the anal opening itself, and it is interconnected with the main pelvic muscles—so the anus is the closest erogenous neighbor of the genitals. The anus even contracts rhythmically during orgasm.

The opening of the anus is surrounded by two muscle rings called *sphincters,* both of which operate independently. The external sphincter is controlled by the central nervous system, so you can tense and relax this sphincter whenever you want. The internal sphincter, however, is controlled by the autonomic part of the nervous system, so it reacts and responds to fear and anxiety during anal sex by tightening up.

The keys to safer and satisfying anal enjoyment are making sure the anus is relaxed before inserting any objects and using copious amounts of lubrication, since the anus is not self-lubricating.

For a comprehensive guide to anal sex, I highly recommend Jack Morin's *Anal Pleasure & Health* and Tristan Taramino's *Ultimate Guide to Anal Sex for Women.*

Safer Anal Play

The same rules do not apply for anal penetration as for vaginal penetration. Although both the vagina and the rectum are lined with soft tissue and are capable of expanding, they are completely dissimilar. The rectum is not straight. After the short canal that connects the anal opening to the rectum, the rectum tilts toward the front of the body. A few inches in, it curves back; then, after a few more inches, it reverses to go forward again.

You can reduce the risk of physical injury during anal penetration by adhering to the following guidelines:

- If it is painful, *stop.*
- Never use force during insertion.
- Avoid using substances that may numb or artificially mask any pain.
- Use lots and lots of lubricant!

Gonorrhea, syphilis, herpes, and human papillomavirus can be transmitted anally. Intestinal parasites, bacteria, or tiny bugs are usually passed along if fecal matter finds its way into someone's mouth or vagina, most likely through oral-anal contact (rimming). Rimming should always involve the use of a latex barrier like a dental dam. If you are fingering the anus, wash your hands or use gloves if moving from anus to vagina. HIV can pass from the semen or blood of an infected person to the bloodstream of a partner through a break in the rectal tissue during anal intercourse. Those who do enjoy anal intercourse should always use a condom.

Kinky Pleasures

As with much of sexuality, there's no universal definition of what is straight, narrow, or off-the-road kinky sexual behavior. True, there are laws about sex acts, and what's considered legal in New York may get you arrested in Tennessee; but in general, words like "kinky" are culturally and socially defined. One person exalts in the beauty that is Michelangelo's *David,* while another person petitions for a loincloth to cover his genitals.

What does it all mean? Basically, if you're into bondage, spanking, fetish, or swinging, you are not alone. A fair number of people link their sexuality to a *paraphilia,* a mental health term used to describe sexual arousal in response to sexual objects or situations that are not part of what is considered "typical" societal arousal and activity patterns. Some people object to the term *paraphilia* because it refers to behaviors that can be engaged in consensually and are not harmful to the participants, but it also refers to illegal and harmful activities like pedophilia. Following are some common paraphilias:*

---

* From the *Diagnostic and Statistical Manual of the American Psychological Association* IV.

- Exhibitionism: deriving sexual pleasure from being watched.
- Fetishism: sexual attraction to particular objects (such as shoes, items of clothing, or body parts).
- Frotteurism: deriving sexual pleasure from rubbing against other people.
- Masochism: deriving sexual pleasure from receiving pain and suffering.
- Sadism: deriving sexual pleasure from inflicting pain and suffering.
- Voyeurism: deriving sexual pleasure from watching others.
- Urophilia: sexual arousal from contact with urine.
- Narratophilia: need to listen to erotic narratives in order to achieve sexual arousal.
- Pictophilia: being dependent on sexy pictures for sexual response.
- Troilism: two people engaged in sexual activities while a third observes.

Most of these activities are harmless unless done without consent, which means mutual agreement. For example, it is perfectly fine to attend a "clothing optional" party, but it's not okay to show up at Uncle Harry and Aunt Edna's sixtieth anniversary part wearing only a leather-studded cock ring.

There is nothing sick or wrong with being kinky, and there are lots of healthy ways to express desires that do not infringe on anyone else's rights. There is a large *S/M* (*sadism and masochism*) community in the United States that focuses on practicing S/M that is *safe, sane*, and *consensual*.

There are organizations, many of which have a presence on the Internet, that can provide information and regional contacts for support and play groups around the country (see resource section for more information).

"I was with a girl who liked to be choked throughout sex. But once while we were doing this she had an asthma attack. It was consensual, but I was terrified about how it would look if something terrible happened, and I had visions of having to call her parents and explain." Sam, twenty-seven.

"I was with a guy who was into golden showers. I thought it was pretty gross to pee on him, but we actually came up with a compromise—we would do it in the shower. That way I didn't feel so nasty and he got what he wanted." Alicia, twenty-three.

"Once this girl I was with asked if she could dress me up in her underwear and put makeup on me. I would never have thought of it myself, but she made it sound really sexy. She ended up taking a bunch of pictures of me, and now I am really nervous that somehow they will end up on the Internet. I will have to plead Halloween costume if that happened!" Reuben, thirty.

"I was on a flight with a boyfriend from New York to Montreal. That's only about an hour long, but he kept on bugging me to have sex in the bathroom. I was saying no, no, but finally I said okay, and he seemed really surprised. So we went to the bathroom, and he was totally freaked out about his bare ass touching the dirty metal toilet seat. I actually got really turned on in the end, and he wasn't so into it." Sasha, twenty-seven.

"I used to date this guy who had a dog named Kona, a keeshond. This dog loved to lick my pussy after sex. At first I pushed the dog away, but after a while it became part of our sexual ritual, and it actually felt pretty good. I nicknamed him 'Kona the Cooze-hound' 'cause he loved to lick my cooze." Georgia, forty-three.

"I slept with a girl who told me she liked to be spanked during sex. The first time we were together, I saw that she had a handprint tattooed on her ass. That was such a turn-on." Dan, thirty-one.

Maybe Dan should meet Arlene, a forty-eight-year-old who also likes spanking, particularly "right as I am about to come and during orgasm."

Cybersex

$\mathcal{S}$peaking of places to travel, I'd be remiss if I didn't mention roaming through cyberspace as part of a phantasmagoric experience. Cyberspace is one place where people feel less inhibited and bolder in asserting their sexuality because of the anonymity (but be careful, you are not always anonymous, and anywhere you travel on the Web you leave a history behind on your computer), which enables you to try out different names, gender identities, sexual preferences, and so on.

Cyberring is actually one of the safest ways around to have sex. Think about it—a totally bodily fluid–free, anonymous way to explore your fantasy. No risk of pregnancy or infections! Of course, it is wise to take precautions if you choose to have encounters, and never give out your name, contact information, or identifying characteristics to the stranger on the other side of the screen. Here is one tale that speaks to the erotic potential of the Internet and its potential for misuse:

"When I was ten years old, my mother finally convinced my father to shell out a couple thousand dollars for a computer. She hooked up AOL, and I promptly began spending late night sessions observing the action in chat rooms entitled 'XXXGirlsneeded.' I believe I still remember the description I gave all those '21-year-old, 6'1", 190-lb. built' fellows. I was '18/f/nyc. Long brown hair, green eyes. About 5'2", 110 pounds, 34C.' The guys always replied with 'u sound hott,' or 'u r so sexie,' or something equally agrammatical. They proceeded to start cybersexing me up. By the time they'd removed my 'shirt' (come to think of it, I was often just wearing my robe for these guys), I'd blocked them and reported them to AOL. I wasn't turned on by this, nor was I trying to be a Good Samaritan. I was just . . . exploring? My mother was open with me about sex. I understood it. I had read plenty of articles in teen magazines about crazy pervs. I knew these guys were crazy pervs. But there's something about it . . . it was the equivalent of a ten-year-old

boy's flipping through his father's stack of Playboys. *It's not yet attractive but seems a clue of what's to come. Of course, those boys invariably miss out on the bunny dating train, and I ended up a homosexual. Make of that what you will."* BVD, twenty-three.

You can find Web sites devoted to just about any sexual practice known to humankind. Just plug the appropriate keywords into your browser (such as Google or Yahoo!), hit "enter," and you will be inundated with Web sites from which to choose. For example, plugging the words *lesbian erotica* into Google returned 4,140,000 results. Click on one to be transported into a seemingly endless array of stories, pictures, and postings. Often these Web sites have discussion sections where you can "chat" with others or post your thoughts, ideas, and opinions. Whether you just read or participate in these discussions is up to you.

A caveat: Recently, a series of articles has been written by experts about the proliferation of cyberporn and its negative effect on sexuality. There are concerns that the easy access and increasing consumption of Internet pornography is coloring relationships, reshaping expectations about sex and body image, and altering how people learn about sex. They report that men (I would add women, too) who frequent porn may develop unrealistic expectations of women's appearance and sexual behavior, have difficulty forming healthy relationships, and be less satisfied sexually. It's food for thought. If you find that you or someone with whom you're involved is developing a compulsive porn habit that disrupts your daily life and interferes with your interpersonal relationships, you may wish to seek help.*

---

* See "For Help and Guidance," page 262.

Toyland

𝒯he joy of toys! I remember the thrill of opening my first Easy-Bake oven; I really, really wanted it and finally got one for my birthday. It helped me learn (who knew that you could cook with a light bulb?), inspired my creativity (decorating those luscious cakes), allowed me to socialize with others (inviting friends over to partake in an Easy-Bake-Off), and provided endless hours of entertainment.

Sex toys, toys for grown-ups, can arouse the same type of enthusiasm. Designed to inspire, delight, and augment pleasure, they are not indicative of your failure as a sexual diva or devo. Think about all the devices we use for technical assistance to enhance our lives—blow dryers, washing machines and dishwashers, automatic toothbrushes, Swiffers, razors. Think about how we entertain ourselves by watching television, listening to CDs, and playing video games. Well, sex toys combine the best of both technical assistance and entertainment pleasure. "It's not normal," you say? "I shouldn't need one," you opine? "Sex should be natural," you assert? "Bull doggy," I say.

Unfortunately, I am not a lawmaker in Texas or Georgia, where as of this printing it is illegal to sell or buy sex toys. Laws like this just show how deep a fear this society has of giving sex play a little boost. So if you are one of the many people who are wary of using sex toys—maybe you are embarrassed, maybe you think you or you partner should be able to bring you to climax unaided, maybe your religion posits that sex toys are wrong, or maybe the thought of stepping into a sleazy sex shop sends shudders down your spine—you might want to reconsider your stance. As we've discussed throughout this book, there is no right way to express your sexuality. Plenty of people enjoy sex toys, whether "singleton," as Bridget Jones likes to say, or in a casual or committed relationship. Now, join me in a walk down the proverbial toy aisle.

Vibrators

First stop, vibrators. Vibrators are the most common sex toy and are available in a wide variety of styles. Some are made of hard, firm plastic. Others feel more rubbery and lifelike. Some buzz contentedly at one speed, while others click busily through multiple settings. There are even vibrators not originally designed for sexual pleasure—but humans are crafty, and it doesn't take a graduate degree to realize that the rhythmic thumping and whirring of your handheld back massager could also do the trick on other body parts. A lot of preorgasmic women actually have their first climax with the help of a vibrator. Betty Dodson, queen of masturbation and author of *Sex for One,* sings their praises. Vibrating is not for women only; the clitoris does not have the market cornered on these pleasure tools. Men enjoy a good vibe now and then, particularly on their perineum.

Dildos

A dildo is a toy that is shaped like a *phallus* (think Washington Monument, cigars, or any other penislike structure). They can be used externally or internally, vaginally, anally, or orally. Some people use dildos for masturbation. Others use dildos with partners. Dildos can be worn in a harness as a "strap-on," or they can be handheld. Women who want to penetrate a male partner orally or anally may use dildos, as might women who are involved with other women. Dildos are also a good tool for men who do not have erections but want to experience penetration with a partner.

Butt Plugs

Another popular toy is the butt plug. Often shaped like a little Christmas tree, a butt plug is designed for just that, plugging your butt. To be more accurate, the butt plug is inserted into the anus. Unlike a dildo, butt plugs usually stay in place and are designed to increase the sensation of fullness. Many people enjoy the feeling of a butt plug being inserted and the sensation of the anal sphincters opening and closing around the toy. Anyone with an anus (that means you!) can enjoy an anal toy. Here are a few tips for using toys with the anus:

- Never use a toy that could slip inside the body. Toys should have a wide flared base or sturdy cord.
- Always use artificial lubricants with an anal toy. The anus does not produce enough lubrication necessary for safe and comfortable anal play.
- Once a toy has been in the anus, do not insert it in the vagina or put it in your mouth, because you can pass bacteria from one orifice to another.

Sensation and Anticipation Toys

Devices like nipple clamps, restraints, handcuffs, floggers, gags, and blindfolds fall into this category. You can even use readily available household items like a feather duster, masking tape, and that stuffed bear you won at the high school carnival. Sometimes these toys are used in conjunction with a role-play or as part of involvement in a particular scene or subculture.

When using restraints or role-play, it is crucial to have a "safe word," so that you'll know when the other person is no longer okay with what you are doing. A safe word has nothing to do with sex or the scene in which you are involved. Don't pick a word like "stop," which could be misinterpreted during a hot session role-playing a helpless kidnap victim. Words like "grapefruit" or "fire truck" may work—unless, perchance, you're role-playing being rescued from a burning fruit stand.

Playing with Your Toys

Contrary to what your mama may have taught you, the primary rule of toys is: *Thou shalt not share.* Toys, like the humans who use them, can pass infections. If you must share a toy, make sure to cover it with a new latex condom for each partner, and if going from anus to vagina or mouth on the same partner, wash the toy thoroughly. Silicone toys can be boiled, and toys that are made out of other plastics or ones with cords or that use batteries can be washed with antibacterial soap and water.

Mama was right, however, about the second rule of toys: *If you don't take care of your toys, I won't get you any more.* Wash your toy after each use, because dried-up, crusted-over body fluids and lubes can cause problems for both the toy and you. Plus, it's just gross.

ACTIVITY: EROTIC POSSIBILITIES

In the following table, check the box next to the word that best describes your experience with the activities listed. For activities that you have tried, record whether or not you enjoyed the activity, what you enjoyed or did not enjoy, and why, and whether you would want to do it again. For those activities that you want to try or would consider trying, record in the "Barriers/Solutions" column what might get in the way of your trying that activity (for instance, lack of knowledge, unwilling partner, guilt, or shame) and any solutions to those barriers.

	Tried, liked	Tried, didn't like	What did you like or not like about it?	Would try again	Want to try	Maybe	Barriers/Solutions	No way
Penetrative anal sex								
Analingus								
Role-playing								
Fantasy clothing or underwear								
Sex parties								
Bondage								
Domination								
Submission								
Sensation play								
Butt plug								
Dildo								
Strap-on								
Stripping								

	Tried, liked	Tried, didn't like	What did you like or not like about it?	Would try again	Want to try	Maybe	Barriers/Solutions	No way
Using a vibrator								
Group sex								
Watching porn								
Reading porn/erotica								
Receptive anal sex								

For those activities that you have tried but didn't like, but would try again, under what circumstances would you (or what would have to be different in order for you to) enjoy this activity (for example, a different partner, more information, level of comfort)?

_____

_____

_____

In the space below, record any other thoughts, questions, or concerns that you have after doing this exercise.

_____

_____

_____

Chapter 11

LEARNING THE LEXICON

*Improve the Way
You Communicate About Sex*

✳ ✳ ✳

*The capacity to listen to what another person is saying,
to take in both their words and also the meaning which
lies behind the words, is crucial to intimacy. It is a skill that
is at the heart of acknowledging that what is going on
in someone else's inner world matters.*
—Stephanie Dowrick,
Intimacy and Solitude, 1991

*T*aryn, thirty-two, tells us, *"I really hate it when I am having
sex with a guy doggie style and he tries to stick it in my ass
without asking. When that happens I just say, 'This session is over!' "*

Maybe you've decided that your sexploration involves being a
bit more daring in bed—which, as Taryn notes above, definitely
requires communication with your partner—but how the heck
are you going to let your missionary-position-only partner
know that you want to try a little bondage?

Todd, thirty-eight, writes, *"I mean, we've been doing it pretty much missionary style for the past ten years. It's going to blow her mind that I want to try something a little wild. I'm afraid she'll think that I've been having an affair or watching porn and getting 'crazy ideas' and accuse me of being a pervert."*

Well, Todd, she may, but you really have *no idea* what she would think about your desire to be more experimental in bed. Maybe the conversation that you need to have first is the one with *yourself*. Maybe *you* are worried that wanting to do those things makes you a pervert. Ask yourself why you think that way. Is it something in your past? Is it the messages you got about what is perverted? Maybe you have been fantasizing about having an affair. Maybe you have looked at some of the Web sites listed in the resource section of this book. So what? Are you fearful that your partner will reject you because of your requests? This may be difficult to grasp, but even if she rejects your request, she is not rejecting *you*. And wanting to explore is normal and healthy.

In any relationship, there will be times in which your needs and desires do not coincide. One person wants to cuddle when the other wants to be left alone. One person wants to make love when the other is absorbed in a really good mystery novel. One person wants to share what happened at work when the other is tired of listening to people complaining all day long. One person wants changes and the other enjoys the status quo. But as long as we accept this and agree to compromise, then being sexually compatible becomes a lot easier.

In the early stage of a relationship, many people are eager to reveal everything to another person, while others want to present their "best" self and may leave out certain truths or details in order to be accepted by or impress someone. Eventually, everyone begins to see another's inner beauty and flaws and discover that this person is not the perfect partner they imagined. Paradoxically, it may become *more* difficult to share intimate details as you get closer, because you feel vulnerable, afraid, and sure that you

TOP REASONS WHY PEOPLE DON'T TALK ABOUT SEX

- They believe that sex is natural and that talking about it ruins it.
- They think that talking takes the romance out of sex.
- They hold on to the myth that their partner should know what to do without being told.
- They feel awkward or embarrassed talking about it.
- They just want to do it and not stop the action.
- They feel vulnerable and exposed if they express their needs and desires.
- They don't want to hurt someone else's feelings or make the other person feel inadequate.
- Their partner gets defensive if they try to talk about sex.

will be judged. There is also the expectation, often in a long-term relationship, that your spouse/partner should know, without being told, what you want or need. But open communication, trust, and understanding are imperative to a healthy relationship—and great for your functional, happy sex life.

There are plenty of communication styles, and you have to pick the one that works best for you. However, you should know that some styles are more effective at conveying your needs than others. First of all, if you want to be heard, you have to make an effort to also hear your partner. There is a big difference between active and passive listening. Marcus, twenty-five, explains, "Sometimes I try to tell my girlfriend how I am feeling, but she seems distracted and just kind of says, 'Uh-huh, okay, sure,' without really giving any opinions." This is passive listening, and it can be really frustrating. If Marcus's girlfriend were an active listener, she would participate in the conversation. Instead of the uh-huhs, she would ask for clarifications, like "Okay, I get what you are saying" or "What do you mean by that?"

Sometimes people think they are communicating well by asking questions like "Did you have an orgasm?" or "Is it okay if we don't have sex tonight?" Unfortunately, these are yes or no questions that don't leave a lot of room for discussion. "What is the best way to make you have an orgasm?" and "How do you like to be touched?" are better questions because they are open-ended and can leave room for discussion.

Some people find it really tricky to make sexual requests. You might know you need oral sex for fifteen minutes before intercourse in order to come but feel it is not your place to ask for this. It might seem selfish to you. But having your sexual needs met is not selfish, and explicitly telling a partner what you need is a lot kinder than forcing that person to fumble around hoping to hit on what you like by accident. The more specific you can be in your requests, the easier life will be for you and your partner!

Eliza, thirty-four, remembers, *"The first time I told Frank what I liked, I felt so ashamed. It seemed so greedy to tell him to use a vibrator on me and then fuck me. But he was really relieved and actually thanked me for making his job easier!"*

If you are worried about how your partner will react, keep in mind the importance of "I" statements. Don't say, "You never make me come." Instead try "I come a lot easier from being on top than on the bottom; can we try that?" You'll be amazed at the difference transferring a few words to yourself can be!

Sometimes we not only need to give direction, but we may also have to accept criticism. It can be hard to hear that you are doing something another person doesn't like. But in order to improve your sex life, it is really important to swallow your pride and accept that maybe there is something you could do differently.

"One of the toughest things I had to hear was that my boyfriend found me exhausting! I really like hard sex and would always ask him to go harder and harder. One day he stopped in the middle and snapped at me that he couldn't go any faster and maybe I should just get myself

off. It sucked to hear that, but I realized that I was demanding more than he could give physically. So now when I need it really hard we use a dildo." Marcella, twenty-two.

As frustrating as it may be to feel inadequate during a sexual encounter, snapping at a partner during sex is never a good idea. In Marcella's case, it sounds as if this had been something her boyfriend had been thinking about for a while and should have brought up in a nonsexual situation. However, Marcella was able to take the criticism and turn it into something positive.

In general, it is much better to be able to offer criticism with a positive comment as well. It works a lot better to say to a partner over breakfast, "Honey, I love how you give me blow jobs. It feels great that you are so gentle, and you look so sexy doing it. I would love it if you were that gentle when you gave me hand jobs, too."

Suggested Steps

Although there are no "rules" about how to communicate around sex, I will share with you some time-tested suggestions that work for many people:

- Find your personal communication style.
- Understand the risks.
- Practice makes perfect.
- Prepare for the worst-case scenario.
- Find the appropriate time.
- Plunge in and do it.

Find Your Personal Communication Style

Several factors are important to consider when it comes to talking about sex: what you are trying to say to the other person, how you feel about what you are trying to say, what words you use, the meaning of those words, and the context in which you use them.

One of the limits of language is that words can be interpreted differently and can take on different meanings depending upon the context in which they are used. Take the word *sad,* for example. If I tell you that I am sad, do I mean that I am "rainy day stuck inside" sad or "my best friend died" sad or "nothing matters anymore" sad? There's no way you would know unless you probed.

One example is the term *making out.* "Making out is kissing with groping," says Jim, twenty-one. "I think making out is when you kiss with tongue and stroke your partner at the same time," offers Vera, thirty-nine. "When I say I made out with someone, it generally implies we had sex, only I don't like to say that, in case the other person wants to keep it private," says Jon, thirty-two. Jamie, fifteen, offers helpfully that "making out is what people used to call 'hooking up.'" Um, right. Anyhow, when it comes to "making out," everyone has a slightly different definition of what this actually means.

There are endless phrases for sexual activities and a multitude of words for sexual body parts (see chapters 6 and 7 for lists of words), and their meanings are not universal.

Consider, for example, the following statement: "Oh, honey, when you put your _____ [suggested words: penis/dick/woody] into my _____ [suggested words: vagina/pussy/love box], it feels sooo good."

What words might you be comfortable using in that statement? Some words may offend you, or you may feel uncomfortable using them. Let's say you use the word *shlong* but your partner doesn't know what a shlong is (FYI, it's a penis). How is he going to know what to put into your love box? Even words with seemingly straightforward meanings have multiple definitions. Or what if you feel empowered by using the word *cunt* to describe your vulva and vagina, but your partner sees it as a degrading term? How will you reconcile these differences?

There are probably thousands of ways to ask for what you need, and any number of them can work. How can you tell what will work for you? Think about conversations or ways that you have communicated with family members, friends, and colleagues. Do you approach them directly, or do you practice the art of subtlety? Is humor your modus operandi? Do you use different techniques in different situations, or do you have a distinct way of interacting? Read the following and see if any of them typify the communication style you use;

Joanne, thirty-eight, and her husband, Kevin, forty-five, feel more comfortable talking in bed with the lights out. Kevin says, *"It's less intimidating that way. I can say what I want without having to see her. In some ways it's more intimate for us to do it that way."*

Tamara, forty, writes letters expressing what's on her mind: *"I'm more articulate in a letter than in a conversation. Plus, I can rewrite it as many times as I have to so that it comes out right."* Her girlfriend usually responds verbally, and that breaks the ice for further conversation.

Anita, thirty-four, practices with a friend first: *"My friend Sarina is great. She knows my partner and can usually predict how he will react. Practicing takes some of the uncertainty out of it for me. And she gives me encouragement."*

Simon, twenty-six, makes notes: *"My girlfriend knows something is up when I approach her with index cards in my hand. But they help me stay on track, especially if she gets upset or tries to change the subject."*

Gloria, thirty-six, prefers the direct approach: *"I tell it like it is. No holds barred. If I don't like what I see or hear, I let him know. When he hears what is on my mind, he knows exactly what I want him to say or do, how I want it done, and the ever important why he must do it ASAP."*

Understand the Risks

$\mathcal{T}$alking about your needs and desires means taking a risk. Discussing your feelings with someone can make you vulnerable, and you might get hurt. But you may want to ask yourself if it is actually your pride that is standing in the way of you and a much more fulfilling sex life.

"I used to be able to hit on guys only when I was drunk. But then this kind of started to worry me, so I forced myself to ask this guy out from work one day. He was this really cute skateboarder/artist type that totally made my knees go weak (a throwback to thirteen-year-old crushes, I'm sure). Anyhow, he said yes and we went out for dinner, and afterwards I invited him back to my place. He seemed really uncomfortable the whole time, but I thought he was just shy. So I actually said to him, 'Do you want to make out?' He said yes and we kissed for a few minutes. But then he pulled away and said he had to leave. At the door he promised to call me again, but I never heard from him. For a few days I felt kind of pathetic, but it actually taught me that getting rejected was not the worst thing in the world. Sometimes you ask someone out and they aren't into you. But if you don't ask, you will never know. And anyhow, plenty of guys do want to make out with you when you bother to ask—even if you are sober!" Erika, thirty.

If you grew up in a household in which you were discouraged from talking (children should be seen and not heard) or, more disturbingly, were punished for expressing yourself, it is understandable that you are reluctant to talk about what you want or need. You may even fear that all of those suppressed needs when expressed might be enormous or insatiable. It's not a rational fear, and it is one that affects a lot of people.

Many people are afraid of rejection and worry that if they express their sexual needs, a partner will get really turned off or freaked out and leave. Some assume that when people are right for each other they don't need to talk about sex because sex will just naturally be perfect. These people are concerned that talking about sex will imply that they are not compatible with a partner. This really isn't the case, however, and like everything in life, good sex takes work.

Practice Makes Perfect

$\mathscr{P}$reparation is the key to success, and practice is the key to preparation. Rehearse what you are going to say. Talk to the dog or to a mirror, or role-play with a trusted friend. Test out different ways of saying what you want. Write down what you want to say; make notes if you have to. You can use the suggestions in this book as is or adapt them into your own words.

Prepare for the Worst-Case Scenario

$\mathscr{T}$he timing is perfect, you were eloquent and caring in your explanation of what you want, and . . . it doesn't go the way you planned. Maybe he got defensive or angry or misunderstood what you were trying to say. Conversations consist of input and output. You can control your output, but you cannot control input or the way someone interprets what you say. For example, Shannon, twenty-eight, was amazed that John, thirty-six, interpreted her saying "I can't have an orgasm just with oral sex" as "You are a lousy lover."

"With a new partner I try to postpone sexual acts as much as I can before they pressure me too much. The first sexual thing I do is mutual masturbation. The most nerve-racking thing for me about being with a new sex partner is probably my worry that they will not like what I am doing or how I'm doing it. My other biggest fear or concern is the realization that the amount of people I've had sex with has now gone up. My biggest fear with a new partner is when they will leave me." Thomas, twenty-six.

Sometimes you may be reluctant to talk about what's bothering you because you are afraid your partner won't understand or will leave you or will think you're a whiner or get mad and stop talking to you. For every conversation that you plan to have, ask yourself: "What is the worst thing that can happen?"

Any time you initiate a conversation, you run the risk that the other person will not want to have that discussion or may disagree with what you are saying. Before you begin a conversation, decide for yourself what compromises you are willing to make for getting what you are requesting. In other words, what is your bottom line?

Prepare for the worst and you'll usually be pleasantly surprised by the actual outcome. Trust me, if someone leaves you because you ask that he or she get tested for sexually transmitted infections, that person is not worth crying over.

A good tactic is to limit criticisms to one issue per discussion. Saying "I get really turned off when you try to have sex with me without showering, and I wish you would shave your legs more often, and can you please keep it down when you come because the neighbors can hear everything" is a huge pill to swallow. Pick one issue, sandwich it with a compliment, and you will see much better results.

If you keep asking your partner for what you want and he or she ignores your requests, it may be time to examine this relationship or seek professional help. If your partner doesn't care about what you have to say, maybe it's time to end the relationship. If he or she gets defensive or upset when you express your desires, you both could probably use some help with your communication. If you can't get by an impasse on your own, a neutral, experienced third party such as a counselor can help you negotiate the rough spots in your relationship.

It can be a good idea to assess whether you think your relationship is healthy. The international reproductive health organization

Planned Parenthood (www.plannedparenthood.org) lists these six qualities as signs of a healthy relationship:

- Respect
- Trust
- Honesty
- Fairness
- Equality
- Good communication

If you don't think your relationship is providing these things, then you might want to reassess.

Find the Appropriate Time

$\mathcal{T}$alking about what you want is important, so don't sell yourself short. Create optimum conditions for discussing what is on your mind. While you're in the car on the way to your in-laws' house is probably not the best time to discuss your need for him not to lick your ear. When you're drifting off to sleep, neither of you can do justice to a conversation about how you wish she wouldn't get jealous of your work buddies. If he's watching his favorite team play the NCAA finals, there is no way you'll get his undivided attention (maybe during half-time). Maybe you can tell him you want to set up some time to talk. Or wait until the weekend, when you may be more re-laxed. Telling someone you wish he or she would last longer in the sack while the two of you are lying in a sweaty tangle of sheets immediately after sex can be a bit hard to take. Some-times it can be tough to talk about sex out of context. But egos tend to be a little less fragile over the breakfast table than they are just after making what you thought was incredible love to your main squeeze.

Plunge In and Do It

$\mathcal{A}$t some point, you just need to take a deep breath, plunge right in, and have the "conversation."

Given people's differences, it makes sense that one person cannot guess what feels good for a partner, no matter how few or how many other people that person has been with. Ideally, someone will ask you what you like, and you will feel comfortable telling him or her. Note that it is normal to experience a change in desire with time or with different partners or with your mood. Perhaps what you have been doing was good for a while, but lately your partner seems to have gotten lazy. Or you used to love how he always massaged your breasts, but now you want him to spend more time kissing your lips. What he or she is doing may be working for you, but maybe you want more of it—longer or harder or slower.

The two quotes that follow are examples of communication styles that haven't worked.

"If something isn't working physically, I try to guide them with my hand; but if something hurts, I immediately balk and get them away from the area that hurts. I don't usually get my point across well, as rarely does the problem get fixed, unless it's one of not touching a certain spot, in which case I make that abundantly clear. If I am uncomfortable, I just go through with it and then later deal with the depression and anxiety brought on by the discomfort." Ronnie, forty-three.

"My partners have all been more vocal than me. I don't mind making sounds, but sometimes I find that I would fake those sounds to compete with his. My methods of communicating about sex are obviously not received well, since, now that I think about it, I don't believe I've ever had a fully satisfying orgasm, though I have come with other people." Thomas, twenty-five.

This is your opportunity to teach your partner how to improve your sexual experience together. How might you broach the subject? Let's use Kendra as an example.

Kendra has a new partner whose idea of foreplay is to put his palm on her vulva and rub up and down. She doesn't find that a big turn-on. Kendra says, *"The way he rubs me is not enough stimulation for me. I want him to be gentler, take more time, and use his fingers more to explore my vagina. When he rubs directly on my clit, it's uncomfortable. I've tried to guide him with my hand, but he doesn't get it. How do I let him know?"*

Things to Think About

You are offering constructive criticism about your partner's sexual ability—a sensitive topic—and there's a method for doing it well. Always compliment him or her first; offer positive feedback about his or her performance before suggesting the improvement. Be specific about what you want your partner to do. Just saying that you want "more" is not enough. What does "more" mean? Five minutes? Thirty minutes? Devise a system for letting him or her know (verbally or not) when you're satisfied. Use a word, expression, or movement (not slapping his or her hand away, please) that you mutually agree upon will indicate that something is working for you. Allow yourself to give your partner directions for what feels good in that moment. That way you can control the situation, and he or she doesn't have to worry about disappointing you.

Remind your partner that what worked in other relationships may not work in this one. Every man and every woman responds differently. Even an individual's personal desire can shift inexplicably. That's what makes us so interesting.

If you are in a long-term relationship and this is the first time you are discussing this topic, your husband or wife or boyfriend or girlfriend may be startled about your revelation. As far as they're concerned, everything has been fine until now. He or she may be defensive or upset about what you are saying. Allow your partner the opportunity to express what he or she is thinking without getting defensive yourself.

If your partner starts to criticize what you have been doing sexually or tells you that things haven't been so good for him or her, either, respond by saying that you are open to improving— as long as the end result is a better sex life!

Heating Things Up with Erotic Talk

$\mathcal{P}$eople love to hear it when they are doing something right. By asking and listening, you will learn about your partner's favorite sexual activities and fantasies, and once you know what they are, it's fun to incorporate them into whispered "hot talk" during sex.

"I like to call my vulva 'pussy.' I grew up in a 'down there' household, and now I am all about being explicit. I love to tell partners to eat my pussy. It makes me feel so powerful!" Kimberly, twenty-two.

Mark, thirty-four, also likes talking dirty: *"Penis is what I use to go to the bathroom. When I'm with a lover, I love to hear him talk about my cock."*

It's not just about names for body parts, either. A lot of sex talk simply involves telling a partner what you want done:

"Hearing my lover tell me to climb on top of him and ride his pole until he bursts gets me so wet," says Catherine, thirty-eight.

Derek, forty-two, loves to have a partner talk about what he is doing: *"When Lisa says, 'I love how you are licking me' and 'It feels so good to have you inside me,' I get really into it. I love to feel appreciated, and it encourages me to keep going."*

Maggie had a different experience with a boyfriend: *"Colin was mute, and I hated it! He never made a sound, not even a little baby whimper or a moan. I never had any idea when he was going to come or even if he was awake! I asked him to be vocal, but it was totally impossible for him. It really had a bad effect on me, too. Maybe the third or fourth time we slept together, he paused during sex and shushed me! Later he said it reminded him too much of his ex, who was really loud. What a buzz kill."*

There is a great episode of *Sex and the City* where Miranda first learns how to talk during sex. It starts off simply with her saying things like "Now you're kissing my breasts" and "I feel you stroking my thighs" and culminates with a very empowering and vocal orgasm. Making noise during sex and talking about your sex play as it happens is a great way to communicate with your partner about what feels good, find your sexy voice, and use new language that can bring you to places you never thought possible.

ACTIVITY: WORDS

Before you start the next exercise, refer back to the lists of words for penis and vulva from the previous chapters. Bring yourself and the lists to the mirror. Stand in front of the mirror and read the lists aloud. Try to figure out which words sound sexy and natural to you and which get stuck in your throat. If you aren't comfortable with any of them, try to come up with some of your own.

Now fill in the spaces below with words that you like and dislike for the following body parts and activities and answer the questions:

	I like	I dislike	Unsure
Breasts			
Genitals			
Nipples			
Buttocks			
Engage in sexual activity			

	I like	I dislike	Unsure
Oral sex on a vulva			
Oral sex on a penis			
Anal intercourse			
Vaginal intercourse			
Fingering a vulva/ vagina			
Using hand on a penis			
Other activities:			

Sexual words/expressions that really turn me *on* are*:

_____

_____

Sexual words/expressions that really turn me *off* are:

_____

_____

*Adapted from Linda DeVilers's *Love Skills: A Fun, Upbeat Guide to Sex-cessful Relationships* (Aphrodite Media, 2002).

Something sexual that I've never really had a good word or expression to describe is:

_____

_____

Some new terms I'd really enjoy using or hearing are:

_____

_____

Next, practice asking for what you want. Try turning the boring clinical statements below into words you are comfortable saying. Make it spicy, hot, sexy, and realistic. It's okay if you laugh; humor and sex go together like popcorn and movies. Here's one example:

Booooring:
I would like you to insert your penis into my vagina. I will require you to use a prophylactic as I am concerned about unplanned pregnancy and sexually transmitted infection.
More Erotic:
Baby, I need to feel your hard cock in my pussy. Here's a love glove 'cause we don't want any unexpected surprises now, do we?

Now it's your turn:
Booooring:
I would like to perform fellatio on you, but I am concerned that I will not enjoy myself if you ejaculate in my mouth. Please be sure to advise me before you undertake such an endeavor.
Your Version:

_____

_____

_____

Booooring:
Would you like to engage in rear entry copulation? I have heard that it can be quite stimulating for both partners.
Your Version:

_____

_____

Booooring:
I would consider performing cunnilingus on your vulva. But I require the use of a latex dam, as I have oral herpes and am worried about viral skin cell shedding on my lip despite the fact that I am not currently exhibiting a lesion.
Your Version:

_____

_____

_____

Booooring:
I find your appearance quite comely. I am interested in a sexual encounter with you. Are you of the homosexual orientation as well?
Your Version:

_____

_____

Booooring:
I would like to attempt receptive anal sex, but I am concerned about my physical discomfort, as your member is quite large and my anus is not self-lubricating. Shall we start with digital penetration and proceed from there?
Your Version:

_____

_____

_____

ASKING FOR WHAT YOU WANT

Now try writing your own sexual script. Use the page below to write out a sexual encounter in which you ask your partner to do, say, or act in a way that you would like (for instance, acting out a fantasy, touching you in a specific way, setting limits on what you are willing to do). Decide when and where this encounter will happen and what you would like to experience. Imagine you are writing this to share with a partner. You don't have to share it, but you may decide you want to after you see your completed masterpiece.

_____

_____

_____

_____

_____

A journey of a thousand miles
begins with a single step.
—Confucius

About ten years ago my brother and I began a tradition of taking adventure vacations together during summers when we were both between relationships. We have gone white-water rafting in the Grand Canyon, kayaking and camping off the coast of British Columbia, and biking and hiking in Hawaii. Each time we embarked on one of these trips, I felt a mixture of excitement, anticipation, and anxiety. What if I don't like the other people on the trip? What the heck was I thinking when I signed up for this? What about bears?

Every vacation we took was filled with foibles, yet fascinating nonetheless, and each excursion renewed my appreciation for nature's beauty, my sense of self, and my place in the world, as well as (one time, at least) my fear and reverence for bears. I always returned home with memories and experiences that changed me. Whether in large, visible ways or small, imperceptible ways, they made me a better person. In a similar way, I hope that this book has encouraged you to explore your own body and desires and in doing so, facilitated change and growth in you.

Understanding how your past affects your sexuality and expanding your way of thinking about sex opens you up to new experiences. These experiences, in turn, are your opportunity to examine your needs and desires and to learn more about your body's capacity for pleasure. If you are committed to continuing that exploration, then you are on the right path toward feeling truly great in bed. Whatever that means for you.

Don't think of this chapter so much as "The End of the Book," but more as the beginning of the lifelong journey of being a more sexually in-tune person. As you embark on the rest of your journey, I encourage you to go off on detours, take the road less traveled, follow your own path, and make pit stops for refueling. I wish you human fumblings, pleasurable moments, physical closeness, emotional intimacy, a range of experiences, courage to take risks, hotness, wetness, and silliness. Enjoy the journey without worrying about the destination and applaud progress, not perfection. As time, circumstance, and partners change, prepare yourself to uncover new and challenging aspects of your sexuality. Use this book as a guide for those times. Revisit the exercises and reread the stories. Use the resources I've provided for lifelong learning.

Bon voyage.

Resources and Other Information

OVERALL GREAT RESOURCES

Books

Guide to Getting It On!, 4th ed., by Paul Joannides (Waldport, Ore.: Goofy Foot Press, 2004)

The New Good Vibrations Guide to Sex by Cathy Winks and Anne Semans (San Francisco, Calif.: Cleis Press, 1997)

Intimacy and Solitude by Stephanie Dowrick (New York: Norton, 1995)

Web Sites

Sexuality Information and Education Council of the United States (SIECUS)

www.siecus.org

National clearinghouse and annotated bibliographies on many sex-related topics and current issues.

Advocates for Youth
www.advocatesforyouth.org/youth/index.htm
> This site includes information on a variety of health and well-being topics, including safer sex, sexually transmitted diseases, healthy relationships, and body image. Materials are available in Spanish, French, and English.

Go Ask Alice
www.goaskalice.columbia.edu
> Nonjudgmental Q&A Web site on a wide variety of sexual health topics written specifically for college students (produced by Columbia University Health Services).

The Kaiser Family Foundation
www.kff.org, www.itsyoursexlife.com

American Association of Sex Educators, Counselors and Therapists
www.aasect.org
> This organization certifies sexuality educators, counselors, and therapists. You can locate a counselor or therapist near you by contacting them.

Planned Parenthood
www.plannedparenthood.org/health
> This site includes information on safer sex, sexually transmitted infections, HIV/AIDS, contraceptives, pregnancy options, and more.

American Social Health Association (ASHA)
www.ashastd.org/stdfaqs/index.html
> This Web site has facts and answers about sexually transmitted infections, including HIV/AIDS, and a sexual health glossary.

National Sexuality Resource Center
www.nsrc.sfsu.edu/Index.cfm
> Clearinghouse for current issues in sexuality, sexuality research, and social policy (affiliated with San Francisco State University).

San Francisco Sex Information
www.sfsi.org
> This site includes frequently asked questions, weekly columns, and access to more information by phone and e-mail.

OTHER RESOURCES

For Women

Sex Matters for Women: A Complete Guide to Taking Care of Your Sexual Self by Sallie Foley, Sally Kope, and Dennis Sugrue (New York: Guilford Press, 2002)

Our Bodies, Ourselves for the New Century by the Boston Women's Health Collective (New York: Simon & Schuster Mail Order, 2005)

Woman: An Intimate Geography by Natalie Angier (New York: Random House/Anchor Books, 2000)
> A wonderful book that celebrates the female body.

A New View of a Woman's Body by the Federation of Feminist Women's Health Centers
> This book captures the diversity and uniqueness of a woman's body through detailed information, images, and illustrations.

For Yourself: The Fulfillment of Female Sexuality by Lonnie Barbach (New York: Penguin Group/Signet, 1975)
   A guide for women who have never had an orgasm or who
   wish to enhance their sexual responsiveness.

Vagina Vérité
www.vaginaverite.com
   This Web site includes questionnaires, articles, links, and information on vagina-related subjects.

For Men

The New Male Sexuality: The Truth About Men, Sex, and Pleasure, rev.
   ed., by Bernie Zilbergeld (New York: Random House, 1999)
*The GMHC Complete Guide to Gay Men's Sexual, Physical and
   Emotional Well-Being: Men Like Us* by Daniel Wolfe (New
   York: Random House, 2000)
The Multi-Orgasmic Male by Mantak Chia and Douglas Abrams
   Arana (San Francisco, Calif.: HarperCollins Publishers/Harper
   SanFrancisco, 1996)

Examining Your Past

*Sex Smart: How Your Childhood Shaped Your Sexual Life and What
   to Do About It* by Aline P. Zoldbrod (Oakland, Calif.: New
   Harbinger Publications, 1998)
Courage to Heal Workbook by Laura Davis (New York: Harper &
   Row, 1990)
   An interactive workbook for male and female survivors of
   child sexual abuse.

Masturbation

Sex for One: The Joy of Self-Loving by Betty Dodson (New York: Crown Publishers/Harmony Press, 1987), www.bettydodson.com

   The penultimate guide to the techniques and pleasures of masturbation from the queen.

Jackin World

www.jackinworld.com

   The ultimate male masturbation resource.

Solo Touch

www.solotouch.com/home.php

   Provides an anonymous forum for discussing masturbation and sexual development, reader-submitted techniques, and other information.

Anal, Oral, and Other Pleasures

Anal Pleasure and Health by Jack Morin (San Francisco, Calif.: Down There Press, 1998)

How to Be a Great Lover by Lou Paget (New York: Random House, 1999)

Let Me Count the Ways: Discovering Great Sex Without Intercourse by Marty Klein and Riki Robbins (New York: Penguin Putnam, 1998)

Ultimate Guide to Anal Sex for Women by Tristan Taormino (San Francisco, Calif.: Cleis Press, 1998)

For Each Other by Lonnie Barbach (New York: Penguin Putnam, 2001)

   How to increase sexual desire, experience orgasms with a partner, and enhance your relationships

Erotica and Porn

The Erotic Mind by Jack Morin (New York: HarperPaperbacks, 1996)

Exhibitionism for the Shy by Carol Queen (San Francisco, Calif.: Down There Press, 1995)

Good Vibrations: The Complete Guide to Vibrators by Joani Blank (San Francisco, Calif.: Down There Press, 1989)

Erotica Readers and Writers Association
www.erotica-readers.com/ERA/index.htm

Sexuality and Aging

Great Sex After 40: Strategies for Lifelong Fulfillment by Marvel L. Williams (New York: John Wiley & Sons, 2000)

Still Doing It: Women and Men over 60 Write About their Sexuality by Joani Blank, ed. (San Francisco, Calif.: Down There Press, 2000)

New Expectations: Sexuality Education for Mid and Later Life by Peggy Brick and Jan Lunquist (New York:SIECUS, 2003)

Older and Wiser: Wit, Wisdom, and Spirited Advice from the Older Generation by Eric W. Johnson (New York: Walker & Co., 1986)

Sexuality and Disability or Illness

Sexual Health Network
www.sexualhealth.com

Provides easy access to sexuality information, education, mutual support, counseling, therapy, health care, products, and other resources for people with disabilities, illness, or natural changes throughout the life cycle and those who love them or care for them.

Awakening Your Sexuality: A Guide for Recovering Women by Stephanie Covington (New York: HarperCollins Publishers, 1991)

Enabling Romance: A Guide to Love, Sex and Relationships for the Disabled by Ken Kroll and Erica Levy Klein (New York: Crown Publishers/Harmony Books, 1992)

Gender and Sexual Orientation

My Gender Workbook: How to Become a Real Man, a Real Woman, the Real You, or Something Else Entirely by Kate Bornstein (New York: Routledge, 1998)

Lesbian Couples: A Guide to Creating Healthy Relationships by D. Merilee Clunis, PhD, and G. Dorsey Green, PhD (Emeryville, Calif.: Seal Press, 2000)
Covers a wide range of topics such as living arrangements, coming out to family and friends, resolving conflict, and understanding each other. Pays special attention to differences in race, class, age, and physical ability.

Love Matters: A Book of Lesbian Romance and Relationships by Linda Sutton, MA (Binghamton, N.Y.: Haworth Press, 1999)
A collection of advice columns and personal reflections.

Growth and Intimacy for Gay Men: A Workbook by Christopher J. Alexander, PhD (Binghamton, N.Y.: Haworth Press, 1997)
A workbook with problem-solving exercises that address subjects such as family, self-image, addiction, dating, relationships, AIDS, and mental health.

Queer Resource Directory
www.qrd.org/qrd
A worldwide directory of queer-related links.

Trans-Health.com
www.trans-health.com
> The online magazine of health and fitness for transsexual and transgendered people.

Bisexual Resource Center
www.biresource.org
> Research and education for the general public and other interested organizations about bisexuality; a support network for individual members of the general public and interested organizations to discuss and obtain information about bisexuality.

The Intersex Society of North America
www.isna.org.
> An education, advocacy, and peer support organization that works to create a world free of shame, secrecy, and unwanted surgery for intersex people.

Gay and Lesbian National Hotline
1-888-THE-GLNH (843-4564)

Sexually Transmitted Infections and Safer Sex

Condomania
www.condomania.com
> Lots of condoms including made-to-fit; everything that is condom, novelty items, games, penis everything, boxers, lubes, and so on.

The Body
www.thebody.com
Comprehensive AIDS and HIV resource site.

STI Referrals
National HPV and Cervical Cancer Resource Center
1-877-HPV-5868

Unspeakable
www.unspeakable.com
A solid site on sexually transmitted infections and diseases.

The National Institutes of Health
www.niaid.nih.gov/publications/stds.htm

Centers for Disease Control and Prevention
www.cdc.gov

Religion and Sexuality

Buddhism, Sexuality, and Gender by Jose Ignacio Cabezón, ed.
   (Albany: State University of New York Press, 1992)
   This book explores diverse social questions as they relate to
   sexual orientation and feminism in the Buddhist world.
Heavenly Sex: Sexuality in the Jewish Tradition by Dr. Ruth K.
   Westheimer and Jonathan Mark (New York: New York
   University Press, 1995)
   This book explores sexuality in the context of Jewish reli-
   gion and culture. It draws a connection between sexuality,
   spirituality, and sexual roles as it examines the books of the
   Bible.
Sexuality: A Reader by Karen Lebacqz with David Sinacore-
   Guinn, ed. (Cleveland, Ohio: Pilgrim Press, 1999)
   This anthology of essays weaves together different dimen-
   sions of sexuality from religious perspectives.
Sexuality and the Black Church: Womanist Perspective by Kelly
   Brown Douglas (Maryknoll, N.Y.: Orbis Books, 1999)

This book addresses why sexuality has been a "taboo" subject for the black church and community.

Working Group on Family Ministries and Human Sexuality
www.ncccusa.org

Raises consciousness in the churches and in society on a variety of sexuality issues.

The Center for Sexuality and Religion
www.ctrsr.org

Establishes the positive relationship between human sexuality and spiritual health by providing clergy and laity with information, education, training, techniques, and skills that foster and advocate the attitudes and values for sexual and spiritual health.

Sex Toys and Other Erotic Adventures

Toys in Babeland
www.babeland.com

Women focused and sex positive; good selection of high-quality toys, books, magazines, videos, harnesses, S/M gear, and educational information.

Good Vibrations
1-800-289-8423 (call for a free catalog)
E-mail:goodvibe@well.com
www.goodvibes.com

Sex-positive shop—does a lot of education; carries high-quality toys, books, videos, educational resources, and so on.

For Help and Guidance

- If the condom breaks or you didn't use protection and are concerned about pregnancy and/or STIs:

Emergency Contraception
Hot line, 1-888-NOT-2-LATE
www.backupyourbirthcontrol.org
> Provides information and referrals to receive emergency contraception from anywhere in the United States.

STI Referrals
National HPV and Cervical Cancer Resource Center
1-877-HPV-5868

- If you are or have been in an unhealthy relationship:

National Domestic Violence Hotlines
1-800-799-SAFE
TTY: 1-800-787-3224
National Bilingual Hotline, 1-800-799-7233

- If you are a survivor of rape or childhood sexual abuse:

Rape, Abuse, and Incest National Network (RAINN)
1-800-656-HOPE
E-mail: RAINNmail@aol.com
National Sexual Assault Bilingual Hotline, 1-800-656-4673

- If you are concerned about sexual addiction:

CybersexualAddiction.com
www.cybersexualaddiction.com
> Offers a self-test, frequently asked questions, and online resources for those with concerns about addiction.

The Society for the Advancement of Sexual Health (SASH)
www.ncsac.org

> Offers hope and valuable resources to those seeking information about sexual addiction. Contains a self-test, referrals to professional and group resources, and frequently asked questions.

✳ Index ✳